HANDBOOK FOR

HOSPITAL SISTERS

BY

FLORENCE S. LEES

SUPERINTENDENT OF THE AMBULANCE OF H. I. & R. H. THE
CROWN PRINCESS OF GERMANY
AND PRUSSIA FOR THE WOUNDED IN THE LATE FRENCH
AND GERMAN WAR.

EDITED BY

HENRY W. ACLAND, M.D., F.R.S.

REGIUS PROFESSOR OF MEDICINE IN THE UNIVERSITY OF
OXFORD, AND
HONORARY PHYSICIAN TO H.R.H. THE PRINCE OF WALES

TO

FLORENCE NIGHTINGALE

THIS BOOK

IS

Dedicated.

PREFACE.

Among the social changes in England during the present century none is more remarkable than the increased desire for systematic care of the sick poor. It is not implied that the humane and religious care of the poor had not been among the chief works of mercy of pious persons generally, and of the religious orders in particular, for centuries past. But since the suppression of the religious orders, and especially since the rapid increase of population produced by our manufactures, it must be allowed that the State has found great difficulty in adequately supplementing the action of private charity towards the sick, and that private charity has been unequal to the task of systematically supplementing the stern economy of the State.

But this period we may hope is passing, and nothing is now more encouraging to philanthropic political economists (for such there are) than the attempts made in every direction to secure such a national organisation as shall reduce to a minimum the preventable sickness among the poor, and reach every needy sufferer, without waste of strength or waste of means.

The present little volume is an attempt to strengthen one corps in that army which is battling with the evils that prey on our great urban populations, or which desolate the rural homes of our agricultural classes.

Completely to appreciate the place of nursing in our body politic needs a little attention. Miss Nightingale first startled this country by making familiar the idea that a cultivated woman of gentle birth could safely leave a wealthy home for the lines of a sickly camp, and staunch the wounds and tend the fevers of an army in the field. She first showed how great a work is here for woman, but at the same time how requisite are training, instruction, and organisation.

Her writings as well as her practice show this. Her "Notes on Nursing," her "Notes on Hospitals," her remarks in the Report of the Cubic Space Commission with respect to nursing in workhouses, her regulations for the Nursing School at St. Thomas's Hospital in London, are but parts of a great landmark she has raised in the history of civilization.

On this landmark there seems to be engraved in clear characters, "NURSING IS THE MEDICAL WORK OF WOMAN."

But the nursing there recorded is an art which needs special mental qualities, special culture, and special power of physical endurance.

Nursing is a department of the profession of Medicine and Surgery.

It is incompatible with the ordinary practice of the physician and the surgeon, because there is often implied entire devotion by the nurse to a single patient, and sometimes, indeed, the devotion to a single patient of two or of three nurses.

Nursing has, therefore, become a special subject of education, and the appliances of the Nursing School also are special.

This is at once seen by considering the work that must be daily done in a large hospital ward—

1st. The common work of cleaning, "housemaid's work." This in a room where there are twenty to thirty sick persons must obviously be constant and laborious if the condition of absolute cleanliness is to be maintained in person and bed, in all articles of furniture, and all the vessels and apparatus of whatever kind for daily use.

2ndly. The work of tending the sick themselves in every variety and complication of disease. Wounds to be dressed, posture to be attended to, medicine to be administered, tempers to be soothed, inquiries wisely answered—directions on all these subjects to be received from the physicians and the surgeons with respect to every one, and to be understood, remembered, and acted on, day by day, week by week, the beds never empty, cure or death removing one anxious charge only to be replaced by another—all these demand no light attention, no feeble character.

3rdly. The work of the one organising mind which is to superintend and regulate the steady harmonious action of one or of several such wards.

The functions, therefore, of a completely skilled nurse are threefold—superintendence, ministration, housework.

The three are distinct only in large institutions. The three must be taught in any complete training institution.

It is the main object of this Treatise to pourtray the proper functions of the skilled nurse—of one who is conversant with all the needs of a ward, is capable of doing all the work, and so of instructing and superintending learners.

It is much to be desired that this subject should be fully understood by the managers of the many hospitals, rate-supported or voluntary, which now exist in every part of the country.

This is not the place for entering at length on the whole question of the relation of "Nursing" to other arrangements connected with national and personal health. It would be unjust, however, both to the author of this Manual and to the reader to omit all allusion to that complex subject.

The "progress of civilization" in this country is bringing about a general revision of the external and obvious arrangements which were supposed to constitute the framework of society. This appears often in an unexpected manner. Half a century ago nothing was more accepted as true than that bleeding was a *sine quâ non* in pneumonia—that all surgeons were men—that cure was the highest function of the physician. We now admit that bleeding is not essential, that surgeons may be women, that in many things, medical as non-medical, we can prevent what we cannot cure.

Thoughtful persons in every department are asking themselves; in this shuffle of the cards what is the outcome to be desired?

In the matter of nurse training this is certain—that a really skilled nurse in many cases influences at least as much as the physician the result of the illness; that nursing is therefore a fit object for the employment of great practical ability, as for the exercise of high moral qualities; that there is here an outlet for the energies and employment for the tender power and skill of good women of almost every class; that five years or ten years as a nursing sister in a hospital should no more disqualify a young lady for a future and different life than going to the bar for a few years should unfit a man for the life of a country gentleman; that a woman who, having had a good general education; such as women now get, and having gone well and wisely through the discipline of Miss Nightingale's school at St. Thomas's, whatever her destiny in life might be, would adorn it, and prove in the truest sense a blessing to those in whose society she was afterwards placed.

That much is certain. General culture followed by the acquisition of some portions of physical science, and the study of their practical application to the relief of human suffering, the habit of firm though gentle command which a ward sister must acquire, the contact with the administrative arrangements of a great hospital, the interest in the great questions of social organisation which surround the charge of the sick poor, all evoked in a manner essentially belonging to the delicacy and the practical sympathy of woman's character, would make as they have made noble female characters.

If there be any who think that the life here praised is one which cannot give scope to high intellectual attainment, they had better grapple more closely with a few of the material and psychical questions which arise round the sick man's bed. Having so grappled they may find, as wiser men have found before, how much there is that centres in one life and in one death for him that has eyes to see and heart to understand.

If these brief hints be germs of truth, the development of intelligent and skilled nursing as a profession will prove of incalculable benefit—1st, to the sick and the poor, in general; and, 2nd, to women and to the medical profession in particular.

Of the sick and the poor more need not be said. Of women, in relation to the medical profession, just a few words should be added.

The Medical Act of 1858 allows women to be registered as medical practitioners. It makes no provision for the registration of trained nurses, however complete their education, and however great their skill, whether as midwives or nurses.

Many accomplished women might reasonably desire the name as well as the function of superintendents of hospitals, or of ward-sisters, or of nurses. At present they can have no such legal recognition of their qualifications in either department, as is obtained by sisters who become school-mistresses, or who are students and teachers of Art. That this ought to be remedied can hardly admit of doubt; but it rests with the women of England to decide whether what is here advocated has their support as well as their approval: or whether the sole relation they will have to the medical profession is to be that of the ordinary licence to practise surgery and medicine as with men. There are signs that some who desire this last, undervalue or despise the profession of nursing in the wide sense of this volume. If these even consulted their own interests they would support and not look down upon what in their view is at all events half way to a higher end.

One remark only as to the training schools. In every county where there is a good hospital some effort should be made for teaching nurses, and for the maintenance of a nursing staff for use in the district. As the sanitary organisation of the counties is made complete, the hospitals, whether rate-supported or voluntary, will become a more living part of the net-work which furnishes the health statistics of the nation. To these centres pupil-nurses and teachers may and should be generally attached. Dispensing might properly form part of their instruction, as in such districts much of the ordinary dispensing might be done by nurses who had been duly instructed and certificated for the purpose.

Whether this volume will aid the work thus slightly sketched the reader will judge. Of the practical qualifications of the writer there can be no question. Miss Florence Lees has proved herself to be a worthy pupil of Miss Nightingale. Trained at St. Thomas's Hospital, as a probationer and nurse, she has studied and worked in Berlin, Dresden, and Kaiserswerth; afterwards as surgical sister for some months at King's College Hospital, in London; subsequently she examined the hospitals of Holland and Denmark; by the kindness of M. Husson, Director-general of the French Civil Hospitals, she was enabled to undergo further training and have more practice in the Hôtel Dieu, Lariboisière, and Enfant Jesus, and to visit the chief hospitals of Paris, prior to serving under the Sœurs de Charité of St. Vincent de Paul, in the great Military Hospitals of Val-de-Grâce and Vincennes. By the permission of General Lebœuf, the then Minister-of-War, she was enabled to work in every part of these hospitals, and by the constant kindness of M. Michel Lévy, Director of the Val-de-Grâce, her training was rendered a most thorough one, from the kitchen and linen-room to the ward-dressings and the operating theatre.

All this done, it became her lot as her desire, to have sole charge of the second typhus station with the 10th Army Corps before Metz, and to move when that was closed, to the Ambulance for wounded of Her Imperial and Royal Highness the Crown Princess of Germany.

These pages record the chief practical conclusions of such an one. I add only that I trust the book may fall into the hands of the Managers of every hospital, and of the Guardians of every Union, as well as into those of the many cultured women who are unofficially engaged, all over England, in the care of their sick sisters and brethren.

HENRY W. ACLAND.

HANDBOOK FOR
HOSPITAL SISTERS

SECTION I.

GENERAL REMARKS ON NURSING; ON THE QUALIFICATIONS OF NURSES; THE DUTIES OF A WARD SISTER TOWARDS THEM AND TO HER SUPERINTENDENT; AND ON THE BEAUTIFYING OF HER WARDS.

"Il ne suffit pas pour obtenir la guérison d'un malade que le médecin agisse suivant les règles de l'art: il faut aussi qu'il trouve un concours dévoué et intelligent chez les personnes qui l'assistent."—Manuel pour l'Infirmier de Visite, publié par ordre du Ministre de la Guerre. Paris: 1870.

Having been told that I have had unusual opportunities for observing the work of Sisters and Nurses in hospitals, at home and abroad, I have been induced to publish the notes which I made in spare moments, when passing through the course of training, or instruction, at these hospitals. Any one who is at all acquainted with work of this kind, will know how, during the day-time spare moments are rare and precious, and how at night-time the weariness of body acts upon the brain, and urges it to seek repose. I offer this as an excuse for the many imperfections of these notes, imperfections of which I am so deeply sensible, that nothing but the earnest solicitations of one to whom I owe all that I know of hospital work, under whom and by whom I have been trained, could have persuaded me to undertake their publication.

I have given this book the title of "A Handbook for Hospital Sisters," because in England head nurses of wards are so called; and my remarks are principally directed to the duties and qualifications of these. Moreover, although many books have appeared in imitation of the first and well known "Notes on Nursing," none of them have been written for, or adapted to the requirements of, those who have to train others.

The term "Sisters" in hospitals abroad, is applied to the Roman Catholic nurses; the corresponding term for Protestants is "Deaconesses." Of whatever persuasion they may be, they, the Sisters, are obliged in their hospitals to pass through the training of Probationary Nurses. This training abroad is, however, different from that given in St. Thomas's Hospital, and in other schools for nurses in this kingdom; but there are in Germany two, one at Darmstadt, under Princess Louis of Hesse, and one at Carlsruhe under the Grand Duchess of Baden, which are justly celebrated for the perfection of their practical and theoretical teaching.

Neither German Deaconesses, nor French Sisters, receive a training thorough in all respects, but they are taught to keep the wards of the sick, as well as everything in connexion with the sick, except perhaps their persons, clean and in order. I never knew a Deaconess, who washed, or saw washed, the feet of her patients, even when, as was the case during the late war, men came into the wards under their charge and superintendence, who had never had clean socks on for months, nor their feet washed during that time. I have received patients, who had been for several weeks under the charge of Deaconess Sisters, in a state which defies description. Their hair was full of vermin, their feet were encrusted with dirt, and if wounded men, the wounds were dressed only superficially. In fever cases, the lips, teeth, and gums were covered with a thick crust (sordes) which had been left on for days.

With French Sisters this never happened; but, on the other hand, a patient, from feelings of false delicacy, would often be left even by them in the most pitiable condition, unless a male Nurse (Infirmier) was within call, to cleanse and arrange him.

Every trained English Nurse knows that all things can be done for a patient "decently and in order;" and indeed, the chief part of the training consists in learning how this should be done. During the late war I had charge of an ambulance for typhus fever, in which there were but few of those articles for the comfort and well-being of the sick, which would in England be considered indispensable, and the number of attendants allowed was of the scantiest. Here the absolute necessity of a previous training was manifest, for I had to do many things for the sick, which in an English hospital could never fall to the lot of any Nurse. Once, one of the poor fellows, who was sensible, said, "Ah, Sister, I do not like that you should do such things for us, but God will reward you." I felt then that I was already rewarded; for what I had dreaded most of all was lest those who were not in delirium, or utterly helpless, should say anything to make my work harder than it already was.

The dread was without foundation; and yet I do not know what I could or should have done in many cases, had it not been for the very practical training I received as a Nightingale probationer in St. Thomas's Hospital, when it was at Newington.

During the late war, many ladies were most eager to go out and nurse the sick and wounded, wishing and expecting to learn nursing in a few lessons, but this knowledge cannot be acquired in a few weeks, or even a few months. A year's training only lays the foundation for the work of the lifetime which is to succeed it.

An old nurse once said to me, (she was then over seventy years of age, and had served in the Crimea under Miss Nightingale,) "it seems to me that the training is never finished; every day I learn something fresh, or see that I ought to learn it." Those ladies, therefore, were mistaken, who thought a mere desire to help, and a willingness to do what they were told, were the only things necessary to make them valuable assistants to over-worked medical men, who had neither time nor inclination to train those under them.

Dr. Gordon The Deputy-Inspector General, Dr. Gordon, who was sent out by the War Office to the siege of Paris, laid special stress on this point, and said that although he would most willingly accord all praise and honour to the ladies who devoted their time and labour to the sick and wounded in Paris, yet he must venture to remark "that there are numerous circumstances in connection with a state of war, which indicate very clearly the existence of an urgent necessity that military hospital organization should be complete, and consist entirely of persons capable of withstanding the discomforts and fatigue inseparable from war.

"The duty of attending upon the sick and wounded is one of vast importance, involving as it often does, the issues of life and death, and therefore so long as the life of an individual holds that importance to himself and to society which our civilization accords to it, the necessity is paramount of attaining the best security possible against its loss."

No one but a woman can give those thousand and one little cares and attentions, which soften the anguish of suffering and disease; and no one but a *nurse* can know what cares and attentions are best to bestow, nor how to bestow them.

The qualifications which are required in a nurse are stated at the head of each paper given to the pupils in our Training Schools; they are—

Cleanliness.	Sobriety.	Punctuality.
Neatness.	Truthfulness.	Trustworthiness.
Obedience.	Honesty.	Quickness and Orderliness.

And she is to be patient, cheerful, and kindly.

And these qualities the Sister must not only exhibit in her own person, but (which is a much harder task) must endeavour to cultivate them in those who are placed under her. I know of no harder task, nor one requiring more Christian love and charity to fulfil it aright. It is easy to get through one's ordinary routine of duties, but it is sometimes very difficult to make nurses and probationers fulfil theirs. If a sister sees that a nurse really tries to remember and obey the orders which she has received, she will do well to have patience with her for a time, however dull she may be, and merely look carefully over her work. I have known a nurse told morning after morning not to forget "that oiled paper or oil-silk were to be placed over the linseed-poultices of her patients;" and yet, so little reliance could be placed upon her doing exactly as she was ordered, that the sister herself, after the dressings were finished, had to examine every poultice, to see that the oil silk had not been omitted.

In our nursing-schools, none but women whose character is above reproach are ever admitted, and therefore upon this point remark is little needed; but the sister should insist that in the wards, and more particularly in a male ward, no immodest jest should be uttered. The nurse should remember that men are keen observers, and quickly detect even the semblance of levity in a woman. Without this watchfulness over the behaviour, a nurse in a male ward will lose that moral influence which she should possess over her charges, and wanting this, no woman is worthy of the name or of the profession of a nurse.

Personal cleanliness, though always insisted upon in our training-schools, is only superficially carried out. I have known nurses whose hair was kept in the most disgraceful condition, with the exception of the little in front that was shown.

A sister should, by example and precept, urge her nurses to take a cold sponging bath every morning, and thoroughly to wash themselves with warm water at night.

All nurses, before the arrival of the chief surgeon for the visit, 'clean themselves,' as they term it; but this cleansing is only for the outward eye, and does not, even in their own phraseology, come under the heading of "a good wash;" the latter treat being reserved for Saturday night or Sunday morning.

Nor, as a rule, does a nurse change her linen frequently enough. I do not see why it should be impossible to provide nurses with their underlinen as well as their outer dress. This is the custom in the hospitals abroad, and the advantages are too obvious to need my dilating on them. Under this rule, and by no other plan, would a sister be able to ensure that her nurses changed their linen, entirely, twice a week; and no nurse should do so less frequently.

It is sometimes difficult to impress upon nurses the necessity of neatness in their own persons, more especially with regard to the arrangement of their hair.

No sister should ever allow a nurse under her charge to wear her hair low down upon her neck behind, or with frisettes or pads of any kind.

The office of nurse is too high and holy an one for any woman called to it to wish to devote much time to the adornment of her person. Her one object as regards herself should be to be clean, simple, and neat, with nothing in her person or attire to attract notice or remark.

In most of our nursing-schools a uniform dress is provided, and ornaments of any kind are strictly forbidden, therefore it is unnecessary to dwell further upon this subject.

Where no special dress or uniform has been yet adopted, I would recommend the brown holland or linen "wrapper," worn by the nurses in the ambulance of the Crown Princess at Homburg. It was buttoned down the front, and could be worn over any dress, and changed in a minute. The ladies and nurses of the Dutch ambulance at Saarbrücken wore dresses and aprons of the same material, but of coarser texture, bound and trimmed with scarlet woollen braid, about half-an-inch wide, which had a bright and pretty effect.

A uniform dress in hospital life is a point of no little importance.

It would be better if a sister paid more attention to the cleanliness of a nurse's apron than is usually done.

A nurse should not be allowed to serve the dinners of the patients wearing the same apron as when she dressed wounds, &c.; she should be provided with a coarse linen apron to be tied over the other, and used only during the distribution of food.

Further, a nurse or probationer should not be allowed to appear at her meals in the apron which she has worn in the wards; she should be provided with an apron of some dark material, which she should be required to wear when "off duty," putting it on immediately upon leaving, and off when entering the wards. For this purpose I should recommend dark blue cotton or linen, or black alpaca.

All hospital aprons should be made nearly large enough to go round the dress, with a large "bib," or square, in front. This pattern is universally worn by Sœurs Hospitalières abroad, and I have heard much ridicule on the subject of the "lady-like" apron worn by sisters and nurses in England, which are certainly more for effect than protection.

I would also recommend loose sleeves of white linen, or of the same material as the dress, if that material can be washed; they should be drawn over the other sleeves, and tied above the elbow during the active duties of the ward.

They should not be worn outside the ward at any time.

A nurse must receive the strictest possible training upon the necessity of method and order. It is essential, not only that she herself should know where to lay her hand on a thing at a moment's notice, but that others should know it also. A "nurse's cupboard," as it is called, is usually a confused mass of bandages, linen, splints, pads, pots of ointment, &c., put there in what she calls "order," but which would never be so termed in any hospital abroad.

If it be permitted, the sister of a ward should have the doors of the nurse's cupboard made of glass, as she can then see that only such things are put in it as require to be kept free from dust, and that splints, air-cushions, and the like, are on a distinct shelf, where the air may pass freely round and above them.

Linen should be kept on a second shelf in the cupboard, and should be arranged in rolls of various sizes: another shelf should be reserved for prepared pads and splints; and another for oilsilk, gutta percha, thread, pins; another for catheters, and other small articles, each of which is to be placed by itself, distinct from the other contents. A fifth shelf or drawer should contain bandages alone, arranged in order according to size.

Every shelf ought to have a label neatly gummed on its edge, naming its contents.

On no pretence should any soiled pad be admitted amongst the others; it should be at once unpicked, and sent to the laundry to be washed and remade.

All greasy preparations for dressings should be kept in neat jars with lids, and should stand on the table where bottles of various medicines are usually kept in store.

The sister should pay special attention to the keeping of these jars and bottles in the most perfect order and cleanliness; and should see that the adhesive labels (where such are used) are replaced by fresh ones when soiled or defaced.

Often a sister will have great trouble in preventing her nurses falling into slow, dawdling habits. I have found more trouble in making nurses finish their work efficiently in a given time, than in almost anything else. A nurse who does not do her work with a certain amount of quickness and precision, will never do it well; for by her lingering too long over one thing, the other parts of her duty suffer.

I have known a nurse give the most painstaking attention to the crockery in the ward, and in consequence leave herself too little time to bestow half the care which was really required for the dressings of the patients. On the other hand, a nurse who wishes to be thought quick, will hurry and bustle everything and everybody in her ward, occasioning much noise and discomfort, without really advancing her work.

The motto of a nurse should be, "Let all things be done decently, and in order." Let her remember that acting on this rule proves that she has been well drilled in her duties, and that she merits the name which she may well be proud of—that of staff-nurse.

That she should be quiet and gentle, is not by any means incompatible with her being quick and active in the discharge of her duties, but is rather a consequence of it.

A nurse whose duties are never performed, or performed ill, has seldom an equable temper, and her patients suffer from her irritability, even when she is of a really kind disposition, and may have chosen her profession because it seemed to present more opportunities than any other vocation in life for exercising that disposition.

A sister must not only note the various habits and characters of her nurses and probationers, but must teach them to be attentive to, and observant of, any change in the patients under their charge. They should be instructed not to allow the slightest alteration in the condition of a patient to escape their notice.

This is of the utmost importance to the comfort and well-being of the sick, more particularly in the cases of those who have lately been operated upon, and of those suffering from fever, small-pox, &c., where it is most necessary that certain symptoms should meet with immediate attention.

A sister always takes pleasure in making her ward look as bright and pleasant as possible; and since Miss Nightingale's appeal on behalf of the sick for flowers and pictures, there are few English hospitals which do not possess one or the other, and therefore I hope a few remarks on the subject may not be out of place.

Strong-smelling flowers should be avoided. Cut flowers should be arranged on the tables in the centre of the ward, so that all the patients may refresh their eyes with them.

Where it is possible, and permitted by the authorities of the hospital, there should be terra-cotta baskets, depending by wires from the ceiling, and filled with trailing German ivy and climbing plants. The effect imparted to a ward by these baskets is well worth the slight expense of first "fixing" them.

I never knew of any plants in a hospital that did not receive the most loving care and attention from both nurses and patients.

In the Nightingale Midwifery Ward, which was formerly at King's College Hospital (but has been removed on account of the mortality resulting from its being attached to a general hospital) there were small round basket-tables, standing in the centre, filled with flowering plants.

In a German institution where I worked for some time, there were pots of long trailing ivy on every window-sill, the effect of which was very good; while the careful washing given to every leaf once a week was great amusement to patients who could do nothing else.

I would venture to remark that pictures in a ward should be as much varied in size and subject as those in a lady's drawing-room.

In some hospitals, where pictures have been allowed, it has been astonishing to observe how the greatest care has been taken to have them of the same height, width, and quality, and to hang them in a straight line all the way round!

Where pictures can be obtained, let them be oil or water-colour paintings, good engravings, photographs, and lithographs; but let those of an inferior type and bad execution be rejected. I do not wish to give a lecture here upon art, but I must add that I consider good pictures valuable not merely in raising the mind, but in actually assisting the recovery.

To conclude these remarks in the words of one whose experience has been greater than that of anyone who has followed her example:— "People say the effect is only on the mind. It is no such thing. The effect is on the body too. Little as we know about the way in which we are affected by form, by colour, and light, we do know this, that they have an actual physical effect. Variety of form and brilliancy of colour in the objects presented to patients are actual means of recovery. A patient can just as much move his leg when it is fractured, as change his thoughts when no external help from variety is given him."

Pictures should be hung with picture wire as in private houses; the two straight pieces of wire, however, should be fastened to two nails, instead of the hooks and rods usual in private houses.

With regard to the choice of pictures, where a sister is consulted, I cannot do better than copy an extract from a paper entitled, "Prints for Cottage Walls":—"They should be drawn from good originals by a masterly hand for the express purpose; not with academic fluency, but with a certain firm, yet tender quaintness, as of the early Italian school, and clearly coloured in strong colour."

A rigid obedience to orders and truthfulness cannot be too strictly enforced. By truthfulness I mean genuine candour, for, as Miss Nightingale remarks, "truth admits of three distinct interpretations," and by one of these a thing may be told in such a way as to give the opposite impression.

A nurse should be taught to state, straightforwardly and honestly, any dereliction of duty, or neglect of orders received. Even at the request of a patient, a nurse must not conceal anything from the sister under whose orders she is placed. The sister is responsible to the doctor for carrying out his orders, and therefore if, through inadvertence or neglect, such orders have been forgotten, the sister must be able to state fully the circumstances of the case.

It is no uncommon thing for the sister of a ward to receive a sharp reprimand from the physician or surgeon, for her nurse's neglect of duty; but it is better a thousand times that she should be unjustly blamed, than that her patient should suffer.

I would here recommend, as a rule without exception, that a nurse should never, under any circumstances, repeat anything of a personal or domestic character with which she may become acquainted, to a patient's friends or relatives. She must be faithful to her trust.

A sister should discourage her nurses talking much to her patients, or of them in their hearing.

I remember once seeing a poor woman in tears, whose general cheerfulness in the ward was almost a proverb. Upon my begging her to say what troubled her, she, with some reluctance, admitted having heard the staff-nurse remark that "there wasn't a single interesting case in the ward! Even 'No. 6' there (herself) wasn't worth the trouble of dressing, for she would probably go out as she came in." And, do what I would, I could never restore the trust and affection with which this nurse had once been regarded by her.

They should regard her as not only their Mistress, but their Mother, or rather Friend in the full sense of the word; as one to whom they could go in any trouble or doubt, being sure of finding sympathy, advice, and help, whether for themselves or others.

They should endeavour to carry out her wishes in the wards, not with grumbling and reluctance, but with a glad and cheerful obedience, which should in itself be a lesson to their nurses and probationers of respect for authority.

The sisters should regard their nurses as their pupils and children, for whom they are responsible, not only to the authorities of the hospital, but to God.

A sister of a ward or division should endeavour to follow one of the rules, common with "sisters" in French hospitals.

Every day she should receive from her nurses a list of such of the patients as are feeble in appetite, or have serious home troubles to add to their own bodily sufferings; and, as far as she can, she should help and comfort them. She should also give a list of the same to the superintendent or matron of the hospital, in order that the latter, in making her daily rounds, may devote special attention to those cases, and consult with the chaplain, how best to lessen that misery with which she has become acquainted.

The daily report to those under their charge Discipline, should be made with all charity, and only grievous cases of misconduct should be reported to the superintendent for reprimand or punishment.

With regard to punishment, I think it would be well in all hospitals if the rule were established, that no nurse or probationer could pass the gates without an order signed by the sister of her ward, mentioning the hours or time during which she might be absent. These orders should be left with the porter at the gate; and upon the return of each nurse, he should add a note, stating precisely at what hour she returned.

Every evening these "orders" should be given in to the superintendent or matron.

Where a nurse had exceeded her time, the matron would desire the sister to inquire into the reasons, and, if necessary, punish the non-observance of rule by reprimand, or by refusing permission to the nurse to leave the hospital, or hospital grounds, on the following day. For a serious cause of offence, however, the matron could forbid her leaving the hospital grounds for a week, or longer, as she might think fit. The matron could occasionally give a longer "leave of absence" to nurses who had especially deserved reward, or whose health seemed to require it. This is often necessary for a nurse who has been long on duty over a painful case.

It must never be forgotten that a well-trained nurse has to be accustomed to military precision, obedience to orders and discipline, and that the "sisters" and "matron" placed over her must enforce attention to these points, while at the same time they must on their side bear in mind the golden rule of charity and love.

It will be impossible but that cases must occur where it is necessary for a sister to reprove a nurse; but I would urge that this should invariably be done in private. A sister may obtain an immense influence for good over her nurses, by letting them see that she is both hurt and grieved by misconduct.

I need not add that a matron or sister should never be guilty of scolding or loud fault-finding in the wards. It will lessen their influence, and it is in every respect objectionable and injurious to nurses and patients.

By such rules alone can a superintendent or sister carry out aright her "charge," both in regard to those under her, and also to her patients.

I cannot do better than conclude this section by transcribing the words of the lady to whom the foundation of the first training-school for nurses in England is due. "To be 'in charge' is certainly not only to carry out the proper measures yourself, but to see that everyone else does so too; to see that no one either wilfully or ignorantly thwarts or prevents such measures. It is neither to do everything yourself, nor to appoint a number of people to each duty, but to ensure that each does that duty to which he is appointed. This is the meaning which must be attached to the word by (above all) those 'in charge' of sick, whether of numbers or of individuals.

"People who are in charge, however, often seem to have a pride in feeling that they will be 'missed,' that no one can understand or carry on their arrangements, their system, books, accounts, &c., but themselves. It seems to me that the pride is rather, carrying on a system in keeping stores, closets, books, accounts, &c., so that anybody can understand and carry them on—so that, in case of absence or illness, one can deliver everything up to others, and know that all will go on as usual, and that one shall never be missed.

"The every-day management of a large ward, let alone of a hospital,—the knowing what are the laws of life and death for men, and what the laws of health for wards—(and wards are healthy or unhealthy, mainly according to the knowledge or ignorance of the nurse)—are not these matters of sufficient importance and difficulty to require learning by experience, and careful inquiry, just as much as any other art?"

SECTION II.

DURATION OF TRAINING REQUIRED TO MAKE SKILLED NURSES OR SUPERINTENDENTS; TRAINING OF THE NIGHTINGALE PROBATIONERS; SUBJECTS IN WHICH NURSES MUST BE SKILFUL.

A probationer's training for a nurse should last one year, but lady probationers or others who are training for duties of superintendence should have, in addition to the first year in nursing duties, a second year of training in the duties of superintendence and household management, including the care of the linen (which is a very essential part of nursing, always committed to the charge of the matron or superintendent), and more advanced theoretical knowledge tested by examination.

To quote Miss Nightingale, "To keep up the spirits, the courage, the activity, the aim at perfection of nurses, they must always be under a superior, who is superior to themselves. . . . I would add what I think important, viz., that a prospect of promotion could thus be held out to all women who entered this profession, not by seniority, but by selection for superior merit and distinguished service, in which length of service could be considered."

Besides the ward training properly so called, there are a number of duties of a medical and surgical character, in which the probationers have to be practically instructed.

This instruction should be given by the resident medical officer at the bedside or otherwise.

St. Thomas's Hospital is the seat of a well-known medical school, several of the teachers attached to which, voluntarily and without remuneration, give lectures to the Nightingale probationers on subjects connected with their special duties, such as elementary instruction in chemistry, with reference to air, water, and food; physiology, with reference to a knowledge of the leading functions of the body; and general instructions on medical and surgical topics.

The ward-sisters are required to keep a weekly record of the progress of the "probationers," and the probationers themselves are required to keep a diary of their ward-work; in which they write day by day an account of their duties.

They are also required to record special cases of disease, injury, or operation, with the daily changes in the case, and the daily alterations in management, such as a nurse ought to know. Besides these books, each probationer keeps notes of the lectures.

They are required to become skilful

(1) In the dressing of blisters, burns, sores, wounds, and in applying fomentations, poultices, and minor dressings.

(2) In the application of leeches, externally and internally.

(3) In the administration of enemas for men and women.

(4) In the management of trusses and appliances in uterine complaints.

(5) In the best method of friction to the body and extremities.

(6) In the management of helpless patients, *i.e.*, moving, changing, personal cleanliness, feeding, keeping warm or cool, preventing and dressing bed-sores managing position.

(7) In bandaging, making bandages, and rollers, lining of splints.

(8) In making the beds of the patients and removing the sheets whilst the patient is in bed.

(9) They are required to attend at operations.

(10) To be competent to cook gruel, arrowroot, egg-flip, puddings, and prepare drinks for the sick.

(11) To understand ventilation, or keeping the ward fresh by night as well as by day; they are to be careful that great cleanliness is observed in all the utensils, those used for the secretions, as well as those required for cooking.

(12) To make strict observations of the sick in the following particulars:—The state of secretions, expectoration, pulse, skin, appetite, intelligence (as delirium or stupor), breathing, sleep, state of wounds, eruptions, formation of matter, effect of diet or of stimulants, and of medicines.

(13) To learn the management of convalescents.

To ensure efficiency, each ward sister should be supplied with a book which corresponds with the list of duties given to the probationers. In a properly constructed ward, each sister might train four probationers.

SECTION III.

ON THE SELECTION OF PROBATIONERS; THE METHOD OF INSTRUCTION RECOMMENDED FOR THE TRAINING OF SKILLED NURSES AND SUPERINTENDENTS; AND SUGGESTIONS WITH REGARD TO EXAMINING AND CERTIFICATING THE SAME.

Every woman applying for admission should be required to fill up the form of application supplied to her by the superintendent of the hospital. Should this and the references given be satisfactory, the superintendent will appoint a day and hour for a preliminary examination.

This should consist of 20 lines of dictation to test writing and spelling.

She should be required to answer at least three questions in each of the following subjects:—

Addition,	Multiplication,
Subtraction,	Division.

Probationers desirous of training for superintendents should be required to write from dictation at least 20 lines on a sheet of fools-cap. A professional subject should be selected.

To answer at least three questions in each of the following subjects:—

Compound	Addition,	Fractions	{ Vulgar,
"	Subtraction		{ Decimal.
"	Multiplication,		
"	Division,		

After admission, every probationer should, if possible, be placed in a surgical ward. Here she should be employed in making the beds, and in the commonest and severest ward duties; spare moments should be devoted to the cutting out and making of bandages, lining of splints, and the like.

She should be permitted to assist the nurse in the making of poultices and the simplest forms of dressings, and in attending to the personal cleanliness and changing of sheets of a patient in bed.

She should also follow the visit, and keep a diary of the duties performed by her.

If the above trial has been satisfactory, the Trial of probationer should now be removed to a medical ward—I say medical, on the supposition that her first month has been passed in a surgical.

The wards should be varied as much as possible.

Here again she should be employed in bedmaking and the commonest and severest ward duties, assisting the nurse in dressings and necessary duties.

She should follow the visit, and keep a diary of the duties performed by her.

If the probationer's conduct has been satisfactory (if not, a longer trial would be required), she should now be sent for one month to the "school," a room in the probationers' part, specially appointed for theoretical instruction.

Here she should be instructed by the sister in charge—

(1) In rapid and correct bandaging, with and without splints.
(2) The names, uses, and appearances of the various surgical instruments and appliances in general use.
(3) The names and position of the chief bones of the human body: the probationer should be encouraged to make drawings of them.
(4) The names and position of the principal arteries, and the mode of arresting hæmorrhage.
(5) The application of trusses, the use of the catheter, bougie, and other appliances.
(6) The use of the thermometer; the abbreviations used in medicine; weights and measures, and their abbreviations.

The sister in charge of the school should at 'the end of the month make a special examination of her pupils as to their knowledge of the above, and test the quickness and beauty of their bandaging by their performance on the "dummy" used for instruction, and on one another.

The names of those competent should be given to the matron or superintendent, who would then appoint them to wards (if possible, surgical), where each probationer should have six patients, simple cases, given her under surveillance, for whom she would be held accountable, *i.e.*, in making their beds, washing, feeding, and the like.

She should be instructed by the nurse how to dress wounds, what to do at operations, and how to prepare patients for the same.

She should daily take notes on her cases, according to the directions given her, and these she should submit to the sister each evening.

She should be instructed by the sister how to give the necessary report to the chief surgeon or physician.

During the 'visit,' the probationer should deliver the report of the sick under her charge to the surgeon or physician, and receive the orders concerning them.

The ward-sister should stand near to correct or remedy any mistake.

After two months satisfactorily passed in a surgical ward, the probationer should now be sent for two months to a medical ward, where she should be placed in charge of four or more different and complicated diseases requiring careful nursing and observation.

The probationer should have entire charge of her cases under the strictest surveillance, with regard to making their beds, preventing bed-sores, personal cleanliness, feeding, keeping warm or cool, &c.

She should be instructed by the sister how to note the temperature, pulse, and respiration of her patients, what observations to make concerning them, and how to give the report to the physician, and follow out his orders.

The sister should stand near the probationer during the visit, to remedy any mistake.

The written report of her cases should be made daily, and given each evening to the sister of the ward.

The absence of "dressings" makes the work in a medical ward lighter than that in a surgical, unless there are many fever cases. The sister will, therefore, have time to instruct her probationers in making gruel, arrow-root, egg-flip, puddings, and drinks for the sick.

Special little delicacies to tempt the appetite, are required for medical cases more than surgical.

The probationer should now be placed on night duty for one month, if possible, in an accident ward. She should receive orders from the sister with regard to special cases; be directed to promote, by noiseless movements, and every other means in her power, the sleep of her patients; to deaden the flare of the fire by throwing ashes on its blaze; and to put coal on the fire without noise, by drawing on a glove and lifting the coal in her hand, or by putting on broken coal in brown-paper bags, made for the purpose.

She should keep an hourly record of the state of her patients, the administering of medicine, food, and stimulants, and the change of dressings. It is a sign that a nurse has done full justice to her training, when she is able to renew the dressing without awakening the patient.

She should be taught to watch and note the least change in the condition of any patient, and be specially alive to any unfavourable signs between the hours of 1 and 4 a.m., when in some maladies there is a particular tendency to failure in the powers of life. During such failure, she should support the powers by suitable food and stimulants, according to the orders given her.

After a month of night duty, the probationer should be placed in sole charge of an operation-case in a private ward. Operation-cases are usually placed in separate wards for one or two weeks, before being moved back into the general ward.

She should be required to write a complete record of the case from the beginning; what treatment has been employed since admission, for the relief of the disease or injury, the nature of the operation, the use or non-use of chloroform, the duration and number of ligatures and sutures used, and the amount of blood lost; if any applications have been made or any appliances used, their nature and mode of employment must be stated; lastly, a daily account of the case must he kept, showing temperature, pulse, appetite, state of the bowels, number of evacuations, their character, if in any way peculiar, colour of urine, and whether there was any deposit, state of the skin, vomiting, complaints of thirst or any pain, and so on, at what hours medicine was given and dressing renewed, and whether the room has been kept at the temperature ordered.

The operator gives directions as to the temperature, which is usually 65° to 70° Fahr., and also whether the air is to be kept moist by having a kettle boiling on the fire, or if it is summer, over a gas flame.

A regular supply of fresh air must be secured, without exposing the patient to a draught.

If the probationer's conduct and her written report on the "case" have been satisfactory, she should now be sent to the Linenry for two or three weeks. Here she would work under the sister in charge, assisting in the arrangement of the linen, old and new, giving and cutting out the same, and stamping and mending things required.

After ten months of practical work and instruction as above, to the satisfaction of the matron or superintendent, the probationer should be sent to the school for the final course of instruction. Here, in common with the other probationers who have passed through the same course of practical instruction, she will receive lectures from teachers appointed for the purpose, on selected portions of

(1) Anatomy.

(2) Physiology.

(3) Pathology.

(4) Chemistry of common life.

(5) On the first dressing of external wounds.

(6) On diet and sick cookery.

Probationers should be required to make notes of these lectures, to be submitted for correction to the sister in charge. The subjects should be varied, and not more than one lecture be given a day.

Each probationer should receive a paper directing a special course of reading; and she should be required, and shown how, to make suitable notes on the books read. The books should bear directly on subjects treated in the course of lectures.

At the end of the two months, completing the year's training, each probationer would have to pass an examination, *vivâ voce* and by written papers, before two or more examiners appointed for that purpose.

She should be examined as to her knowledge of

(1) The human body, including the names and position of the principal arteries, and the mode of arresting hæmorrhage.

(2) Elementary chemistry, with regard to air, water, and food.

(3) The application of fomentations, poultices, mustard plaisters, blisters, leeches, injections.

(4) The making and application of bandages, minor dressings, trusses, and lining splints.

(5) The management of helpless patients as to moving, changing, cleanliness, feeding and administration of medicines.

(6) The names, uses, and appearances of the various surgical instruments and appliances in general use.

(7) The best mode of cleaning ward floors, hospital furniture, and utensils.

(8) The use, and mode of observing and noting the range of meteorological instruments, but more particularly the thermometer, as used for ascertaining the temperature of patients, and the heat of baths.

(9) The method of regulating the ventilation of the wards, and the object of such ventilation.

(10) The observation of the sick, as regards the appetite, intelligence, breathing, sleep, secretions, expectoration, pulse, skin, state of wounds, eruptions, with a view of testing her ability to give an intelligible account of the patient's history between the visits of the medical officer.

(11) The cooking of gruel, arrowroot, egg-flip, puddings, and preparation of drinks, for the sick.

(12) The meaning of the abbreviations used in prescriptions; weights and measures; and the characters generally used for the same in physicians' prescriptions.

According to her abilities, she would then be certificated a 1st or 2nd class nurse, and a suitable appointment found for her.

At the end of two years' active service and satisfactory conduct, in the situation appointed by the matron or authorities of the nursing school, there should be awarded to a

1st Class Nurse,—A silver medal, with "Nurse of 1st class," the name, and stamp or cipher, of the training school in relief on one side; and on the reverse, the engraved name of the nurse to whom it was awarded, and the date.

2nd Class Nurse,—A silver electro-plated medal, with "Nurse of 2nd class," the name, and stamp or cipher of the training school in relief on one side; and on the reverse, the engraved name of the nurse to whom it was awarded, and the date.

Silver electro-plate is preferable to bronze, as it is not desirable that patients should discern between a first and second class nurse.

RULES WITH REGARD TO EXAMINATIONS.

The rules that I propose are:—

I. No probationer should be admitted to the lectures and theoretical course of teaching, unless her practical duties in the wards had been fulfilled to the entire satisfaction of the ward-sisters, and to the matron or superintendent, and unless her general conduct had been good.

II. Any medical officer, who had cause to be dissatisfied with her nursing or attention, should mention it to the sister of the ward, whose duty it would be to see that the faults complained of were remedied.

In case of disobedience or hopeless stupidity, the probationer should be reported by the sister to the matron or superintendent, who would act with regard to her as she thought fit, either by changing her service, or dismissing her from the school.

III. Ladies desirous of qualifying themselves for the office of ward-sisters, or superintendents of hospitals, would be required, in addition to the above year's training and examination, to spend six or twelve months more (according to capacity) in the school. During this time they would be further instructed in household management and superintendence, the care, management, storing, mending, and issuing of the linen; and the art of instructing and training others; the last could be best learnt by their acting as assistants in the training school.

IV. They should be required to go through a special course of reading marked out for them, and to attend a course of lectures, on

Hygiene, and Chemistry or Botany.

A knowledge of one subject in Natural Science, tested by examination, should be held a *sine quâ non* for any one desirous of being a superintendent.

They should be required to have a reasonable knowledge of anatomy, physiology, and the classification of disease.

V. At the end of six months, they must separately pass an examination on the "general duties of superintendence and household management," named in Rule III., before the matron or superintendent, and the head sister of the nursing school.

The fee of £1, exacted from each pupil entering for the examination, should be devoted to the use of the school.

If the examination is satisfactory, a certificate will then be given her, of her having passed, and she will be permitted to enter for the final examination, which will be held by two or more examiners appointed for that purpose.

VI. Each candidate for the final examination should produce her certificate of "general efficiency in management." A fee of £2 would be required from each pupil entering for this examination.

Theoretical knowledge will in this case be tested *vivâ voce* and by written answers.

If successful, she will then receive the 1st or 2nd class medal of a superintendent, and be registered as such at the school, or, if such register be legally recognised, at the office of the General Medical Council.

VII. Unsuccessful candidates are permitted to study for another six months, and enter for a second examination. If they again fail, they must now be dismissed: they may, however, serve, if they themselves desire it, as staff nurses for two years in the situation appointed them, receiving at the end of that time their medals as 1st class Nurses.

VIII. It shall be open to all former certificated 1st class pupils of the school, to enter for the training and examination for superintendent, upon bringing a satisfactory certificate of conduct, and upon payment of the usual sum for board and instruction during their residence.

IX. Medals for superintendents shall be of gold, gilt, and of silver-gilt: 1st Class, shall be of gold, with

> Superintendents' 1st Class medal in the nursing school of "M. or N.," surrounding the cipher or arms of the school on one side, on the reverse side shall be the motto of the said school, and in the centre the engraved name of the recipient, with the date when the medal was given.
>
> 2nd Class, shall be in silver gilt, and in all respects as above, except 2nd instead of 1st.

X. All ladies desirous of becoming superintendents must obtain a *1st class certificate as nurse*, before their names could be entered for the additional training required for superintendents.

It should be open to all nurses of the 2nd class to enter again for the nurses' examination, and try for a 1st class certificate, after two years at least of complete and satisfactory service in the situations found for them. Should they obtain the silver medal of the 1st class, the electro-plated one of the 2nd class ought to be given up to, and retained by, the school authorities.

Where it is possible, I would recommend the connexion of an orphanage with a nursing school. Here arrangements and provisions could be made for girls between the age of fourteen and sixteen, to learn under a proper female head, sick-cookery, cleaning, needle-work orderly habits, all that is learnt in a servant's training school, and to take their turn in doing what they can be taught to do in the children's sick-wards. They could also receive elementary instruction in chemistry and physiology. Girls so trained would make the best nurses.

For orphans of gentle birth, I would recommend that the last year of their studies should be devoted more especially to those subjects which would be required in their examination for superintendents, and that they should also spend three months in learning the sick-cookery, and duties mentioned above.

SECTION IV.

TRAINING OF THE FRENCH INFIRMIERS DE VISITE FOR MILITARY HOSPITALS; COURSE OF INSTRUCTION.

The hospital attendants are both practically and theoretically taught at the Val-de-Grâce. The course of instruction lasts two months: the first is devoted to theoretical teaching, which the students attend in classes: the second month is devoted to practical teaching in the (military) hospital attached to that establishment.

The following is the instruction given in the classes:—

(1) The system of the books, or "cahiers de visite."

(2) How to keep a list of the daily food and medicines ordered to patients.

(3) How to dress and bandage ordinary wounds.

(4) The contents of the waggons attached to the "ambulance" are explained to them.

(5) The best way for raising and removing the wounded.

(6) The applying of "gouttières" to fractured limbs.

(7) The first thing to be done in case of hæmorrhage, viz., compression by hand, by extemporary tourniquet, and plugging.

The practical instruction given in the wards is as follows:—

(1) Keeping the visit-books, or "cahiers de visite."

(2) The daily tables for diet and medicines to be given to patients.

(3) Bandaging and dressing wounds.

DUTIES OF THE "INFIRMIERS DE VISITE," OR HOSPITAL ATTENDANTS.

The hospital attendants have, under the immediate supervision of the surgeons, to keep the visiting-book, and to take care that the medicine which is daily ordered by the surgeons is regularly administered to the patients; they also have to give out the medicines, and make the bandages.

Each hospital attendant on entering has a copy of this manual given to him, and also a small surgical case containing the following:—

> A pair of scissors.   Dressing forceps.
> A razor.   A spatula.

This case, as well as the copy of this manual, is retained by him, and their cost is deducted from his earnings.

Supposing that any of the surgical instruments be lost, the hospital attendants have to replace them at their own expense. The head surgeons at the military hospitals examine the cases at least once a month, and make sure that each has its full equipment, and that each instrument is clean and fit for use.

The hospital attendants are bound to perform the duties which are allotted to them, no matter what they may be. The charge of the visit books they take in turn every alternate month, and make out the totals of the prescriptions, and bandaging.

The chief surgeon and the assistant-surgeons practise the hospital attendants in the art of bandaging, and avail themselves of their assistance in cases not requiring the presence of many surgeons.

The infirmiers have to keep a list of all the bandages, &c, used; count and write down the same for the laundry, and keep them in good order and repair. When the bandages or other linen used in dressings are worn out, or unfit for use, the infirmier is charged to get the same exchanged for new by the steward at the stores.

THEORETICAL COURSE OF INSTRUCTION OF "INFIRMIERS DE VISITE," INTRODUCED ABOUT 1848.

I was present at the Val-de-Grâce whilst this special instruction was being given, and attended regularly the school for infirmiers during this time. It lasted eight weeks, and the pupils consisted of 70 of the most intelligent orderlies who had been working in the wards of the Val-de-Grâce as assistant nurses, or infirmiers, for at least ten months before they were allowed to receive any special theoretical instruction. This was as follows—

> The first fifteen days were occupied in learning abbreviations, signs, and the more common diets or medicines given. At the end of that time, those who were dull, careless, or indolent, were dismissed, and the others only were permitted to remain the rest of the time,

41 days. Any found deficient at the end of that time, were not permitted to pass, and were dismissed altogether. Half of the most intelligent of those who passed were sent to the different Salles, where they followed the visit, and kept a "cahier de visite," making the "relevés" or totals after it, for the Dépense, Pharmacie, and Tisanerie. At the end of the fifteen days, they received their "grade," and the "embroidered collar," &c., and were sent to different hospitals as required, being replaced in the wards by the other half who had now become capable of supplying their place.

They were in the school—a long garret on the top of one of the wards—facing their dormitory, from 7 till 10 o'clock, and from 12 till 4.

The first three days they did nothing but copy incessantly the abbreviations used in medicine. Every list of abbreviations must be copied at least four times. In this manner they learnt the abbreviations by heart.

Afterwards they commenced with a demonstration on the large black board of the manner of writing the quantity of medicine required, the number of patients, and so on, and the signs in most common use to denote what diet they are on; this was succeeded by a dictation of the same. They were now supposed to have become accustomed to the signs used, and step by step the dictation was made more complicated.

The dictations were marked and numbered, Ire Leçon, 2nde Leçon, &c., and were taken in order; they were drawn up by Dr. Meurs, who visited the school every morning for an hour, returning at noon for bandaging, to see that all was done in order, and to inspect the papers.

The papers for these dictations were printed and ruled, as for a "cahier de visite," and were furnished by order of the Minister for War.

The dictation was succeeded by the "relevé," or "total," which each made in silence. The papers were then given in to the sergeant, who corrected them, while the monitors gave a fresh dictation or the same over again.

After the first 15 days they commenced lessons on bandaging. Dr. Meurs explained the principles of bandaging, and showed them once each bandage. The sergeant afterwards showed each bandage again, and impressed the rules for doing the same.

They had about 40 legs (with toes properly defined) in plaster of Paris or wood, which were placed on the tables. Each infirmier must practise for two hours on that and that only, until his bandaging is not only perfectly well done, but done with celerity and according to rule.

The sergeant gave a lesson on living subjects. He took the arm of one of the infirmiers, and bandaged it before them all, over his shirt sleeve. Then each man in turn had to bandage his neighbour, and be bandaged.

The bandage lesson lasted two hours each day.

Dr. Meurs at the end of the month examined them as to their proficiency.

After a month they were taken out to learn how to pack and unpack a "caisse d'ambulance," or cart for hospital stores.

They are expected to become so expert that in seven minutes the "caisse" must be packed, and their coffee made and drunk!

There are certain rules for packing, which they must learn by heart, that they may fetch immediately anything required by the surgeons on a field of battle, without having to open and examine each basket separately.

CAHIERS DE VISITE.

These consist of two books for each "service," that is, for the odd and even numbers.

Each patient has a page to himself, which is numbered for one calendar month, and contains the diet, wine, medicaments, tisane, and any observations the doctor may think well to make on the disease, operation, or otherwise.

At a glance, therefore, you have the history of a patient from the time he has entered the hospital.

There are special marks to denote the regime or diet of each patient, which, however, they say are learnt in three days.

CARRYING THE WOUNDED.

Once a week, for an hour or two, the whole school of orderlies was exercised in lifting and transporting the wounded. One of their number being the wounded, two of the others placed him gently on the canvas stretcher, and then raising it bore him off.

A wooden horse was brought out, and the orderlies were instructed how to fasten a small chair of iron and leather on each side of the curious old pack-saddle, to carry those who were slightly wounded, and then to lift in two wounded men at the same time, that the equilibrium might not be destroyed. The chairs were then removed.

For the more seriously wounded, however, there were long light iron bedsteads, with a canvas sacking, thin light iron rods being pulled over the head to support a canopy, as a shield against sun or rain. Four orderlies were now told off to raise these beds, and hook them to the pack-saddle instead of the seats, and the beds were hung each side of the horse as fairly and evenly as the chairs had been.

SECTION V.

THE LINENRY; AND GENERAL RULES WITH REGARD TO THE CHANGE AND EXCHANGE OF LINEN.

The linen-room should be large, well-lighted, and ventilated, with proper appliances for heating it throughout in winter. The floor, presses, and shelves should be of polished oak, or of stained and polished deal. The scrubbing necessary for deal flooring renders the atmosphere too damp, as linen and woollen goods readily absorb and retain any moisture in the air.

Where the room has windows on both sides, it is best to have the linen presses or racks placed between each window and at right angles to the wall, but leaving a free passage in the middle of the room.

The presses should consist of long shelves, or of racks made of wood, about three inches wide, placed three inches apart from each other.

Shelves should be divided into compartments, according to the linen or woollen goods they are to contain.

Solid shelves should never be permitted in a linen or store-room, as it is necessary that air should freely permeate the whole.

Each shelf or division should have a ticket or label attached to it, stating its contents.

The best labels are made of white polished earthenware or porcelain, with the name distinctly printed on it in black, and containing a small space for inserting a paper or card, having the number of contents written on it.

These numbers sometimes vary, and they can thus be easily changed when required.

The linen sister is responsible for the linenry being kept in good order, and has to see that the articles of bedding and clothing are kept well aired, in good repair, and properly folded, classified, and arranged on the racks or shelves; and that a proper supply of everything is always on hand to meet exchanges, and other demands.

She should make herself thoroughly acquainted with the number, condition, and use of every article in store, in order to make the necessary issues with facility. I would therefore recommend the method of the French sisters in arranging all linen and woollen goods in tens, twenties, or fifties: every alternate piece being arranged in special patterns, "squares," and peaks. It has a pleasing and varied effect, and facilitates the whole.

The sister must see that, all linen and woollen goods are properly marked—stamping the new with name, date, and number, and re-stamping the old when required.

Attached to the linenry should be another and smaller room, for use as a work-room. This should be used for cutting-out and placing new linen, for mending or executing needful repairs, for placing work to be done in the female wards, and for the tearing up of old or condemned linen.

The latter should never be done in the linenry, on account of the dust created.

No ward-sister or nurse should be permitted to enter the linen-room, therefore one end of it should be partitioned off by a long moveable table or counter, on which—or on the other side of which, the fresh linen for each ward or division should be arranged with its cancelled check pinned to it.

On the days for giving out fresh linen, a bell should be rung outside the linenry at the hour appointed by order of the sister, that the ward sisters may not be kept unduly waiting. Each ward-sister, accompanied by one or more of her nurses, will then enter the part of linenry appointed, compare her packet of linen with her check for the same, and cause it to be taken to her ward. She must then deliver up the check to the linen-sister.

To enable each ward-sister to supply changes of linen when required, she should have in her charge a small supply of linen extra to that in actual use in the wards. These articles, with inventory of the same, should be issued to her by the linen sister once a year.

It will be the duty of the linen-sister to keep in a linen store ledger, in which she will enter on the left hand, or debit side, all articles received by her; and on the right hand, or credit side, all articles issued by her for ward, laundry, or other purposes. The ledger should be duly balanced by her on the last day of the month, or oftener, if necessary, to enable her to ascertain whether the stock on hand is correct.

Requisitions for linen, &c., from the linenry should be accompanied by a signed receipt of the person making the demand, for which purpose the usual form of linen check-book for hospital service should be used.

The linen-sister should keep a separate debtor and creditor account with every ward, and every other department of the hospital, and an accurate account of all articles daily received and issued.

The linen-sister, accompanied by one or more of her assistants, will see the separate packets of foul linen from every ward or division counted out before her in the room or place appointed for that purpose.

When the number of any article differs from the check sent with it, they should again be recounted, and where the ward-sisters list is found incorrect, the linen -sister will draw a line with red ink through the number given, and write the correct amount in the same.

If any article be found injured or stained, apparently in consequence of carelessness, or neglect, the linen-sister will mark and lay it on one side, for the inspection of the matron or superintendent.

All ink or other stains, cuts, burns, or deficiencies discovered, should be recorded in her daily note-book for the information of the superintendent.

The superintendent will fine or reprimand the sister or nurse through whose fault the linen has been injured, and, where it is necessary, see that the same is replaced.

The soiled articles should be removed to the laundry or handed over to the laundress who may contract for the same, on the day, or days, appointed, accompanied by a list signed by the linen sister, of the articles so delivered. On this list an acknowledgment should be given by the laundress, after she has carefully inspected and counted the articles delivered, and entered the numbers in her laundry account book.

When washed, the articles should be delivered at the linenry, and a receipt given for the same by the linen-sister.

The linen-sister should count over the articles on their re-delivery, and make a thorough inspection of them, in order to ascertain that the work has been properly performed, and that the various articles, especially sheets and personal linen, are in a dry condition.

She should now divide them into three classes—*i.e.*, good, bad, and indifferent.

(1) Linen in good repair should be put by in the linenry, in the place appointed for the same.

(2) Linen which is condemned as past
repair should be numbered and sent into the work-room, to serve for future repairs, for bandages, or other purposes.

(3) Linen which is numbered "indifferent" should be sent to the workroom, to be mended and put in thorough repair, before being placed in the linenry.

USES OF OLD LINEN.

In English hospitals it is customary for the sister of each ward to make, or see that her nurses and probationers make, the bandages, and lining for splints, &c., required in her ward.

The sister in charge of the linenry must provide her with linen for that purpose, and for compresses and dressings, when required. One day in the week should be appointed for giving out the same. The linen-sister will be careful that no linen is destroyed which can be efficiently repaired for future use, and that sufficient is retained in the workroom for repairing other linen.

Sheets should be torn up into strips about 9½ inches wide, and the length of the sheet; these strips being of different quality and quantity, and numbered 1, 2, 3.

No. 1 should consist of three strips of the best parts of sheets torn up, and be without darns or patches. These should be used for surgical bandages.

No. 2 should consist of two strips of inferior quality, to be used for compresses, lining of splints, &c.

No. 3 should also consist of two strips, but of the oldest and worst part of the sheets destroyed, to be used for medical bandages, blister dressings, poultices, and the like.

Hand-towels and table cloths should be made into "squares," for lithotomy, ophthalmic, and other operation cases.

Old blankets should be cut into squares, numbered, and given out for the scrubber's use, or cleaning purposes.

Cotton curtains and quilts should be made into dusters, marked and numbered.

Round towels should be made into squares, marked and numbered, for knife or "pantry cloths," for use in the wards.

Bed-ticks and bolsters should be made into "dryers" for scrubber's use, and hemmed but not marked.

The linenry of a "general hospital" of 200 beds should contain—

- 500 Sheets (linen).
- 500   "   (cotton).
- 400 Counterpanes.
- 500 Pillow-cases.
- 250 Draw-sheets.
- 800 Blankets.
- 600 Counterpanes.
- 250 Round towels.
- 500 Hand-towels.
- 50 Diaper table-cloths.
- 200 Dusters.
- 50 Pantry or knife-cloths.
- 6 Strait-waistcoats. These are now seldom used, and should never be of the kind which tie behind with long sleeves, as they irritate the patient. They should simply be a belt to go round the waist, with gloves attached for the patient's hands.

Wearing apparel is seldom provided in English hospitals, with the exception of our workhouse infirmaries and military hospitals. It is usual to have twice as many articles of woollen or outward articles of apparel as there are patients, and three times as many articles of under-clothing, socks, and handkerchiefs.

SECTION VI.

DESCRIPTION OF A FRENCH "LINGERIE," OR LINENRY; AND OF A CHAMBRE DE LINGE A PANSEMENT, OR ROOM FOR THE LINEN REQUIRED FOR DRESSINGS.

The *lingerie* is under the superintendence of a ward-sister called la mere (mother—the Augustinian sisters being so termed), assisted by one novice, two women, and two *garçons* or male assistants.

It is a large room, well ventilated, and containing presses for all the linen used in the hospital. The floor is of polished oak. All the stands, steps, counters, &c., are of oak, or of stained and polished wood. On each side of the longest counter, which is in the centre of the room, are presses for linen, formed entirely of pieces of wood about three or four inches wide, with spaces between them of the same width, to admit a free current of air.

From the laundry the linen is sent to the *mère* of the *lingerie* to fold, or see folded. After each article has been separately smoothed by hand and folded, they are put by in packets of fifties or hundreds in the press, and thus by their own weight, are rendered as smooth as if they had been mangled. Each press is divided into 45 compartments for sheets, draw-sheets, &c., and linen for patients, *employés*, nurses, and sisters.

The linen for the sisters is sent up to the convent, as soon as it has been counted and folded. Each sister has her things marked with the first letter of her name, followed by S. for Sœur (*e.g.* U. S. for Ursula, Sœur).

"Employés" receive one pair of sheets a month; also each week two pair of large linen over-sleeves, and sometimes more; two large aprons of white linen, and three (or if required, more) servant's aprons, which are worn by sisters, nurses, and *employés* to cover the former. *Infirmières* , or women nurses, receive also two caps, one dress, and two fichus without starch. *Infirmiers* or male nurses receive one pair of linen trousers and two jackets.

Ward linen is changed every day, excepting Wednesdays and Sundays, the latter day being freer, and the clean things from the wash arriving on the former.

A list of the soiled linen is made out each day by the *mère de la salle* , or ward-sister, and sent down by one of her *garçons*, who waits to see it counted by the women of the linenry, in the *"salle,"* or room for soiled linen. He receives a check for it, which he leaves in the linenry, before returning to his ward. The novice in the linenry places the number of sheets, &c., written on the check, under the name of the ward to which it belongs. Every ward has its name written over a marked space on the wall, down one side of the room, and under this its linen is always arranged, with check attached.

At half-past ten, or a quarter to eleven, the *mère* leaves the *salle* for soiled linen, and on arriving at the linenry recounts the packet from each ward and compares its check with the list sent from the ward.

At eleven o'clock a bell is rung, and a sister from each ward, with one or two assistants, enters the linenry, and going to where the name of her ward is placed, counts over her clean linen, comparing it with the list attached. It is then "packed" on the back of the *garçon* by one of the men, and carried at once to the *salle* to which it belongs. Here it is again re-counted by the *mère* and arranged by her in her linen closet.

In a quarter of an hour the linenry is again quiet; every sister, nurse, and garçon of the wards having disappeared with their linen.

I will give here the lists of linen changed for two wards in the Hôtel-Dieu on a Thursday, *i.e.,* linen required for *two* days:—

S. Lazare; Number of Patients, 40.

Sheets, 177; draw sheets, 95; pillow-cases, 86; dusters, 25.

Salle S. Jeanne; Number of Patients, 82.

Sheets, 300; draw sheets, 250; pillow-cases, 212; dusters, 24.

If a sister of a salle found that she had not enough sheets, &c., in reserve for the days when the linen was not changed—viz., Wednesday and Sunday, she sent a *"bon,"* or check, for the number of things required. These were supplied at once, and deducted from her linen the next day of change. The check being torn up the middle to show that the debt had been paid.

All linen is sent once a week to the Salpêtrière, in charge of one of the women of the linenry, who waits to see it counted by the people there, and obtain a receipt for the same. Every Wednesday it is returned clean, but neither folded nor mangled, in charge of one of the Salpêtrière women, who also remains to see it counted by the sister of the linenry, and obtain a receipt for it, duly signed by her.

When the clean linen is damped and folded, it is separated into three different packets—viz., 1. Good; 2. Requiring mending; and 3. Destruction.

Mending is done at the Salpêtrière, to which also all things appointed for destruction are sent to "mend work," or make into compresses or lint.

Of all "destruction linen," or linen which has been "patched" more than once, a list is carefully made out by the linen-sister, who sends it once in three months to the Salpêtrière, receiving new linen in exchange from the central depot.

The *Cabinet de la mère*, or sitting-room of the linen-sister, is a pretty little room adjoining the linenry, with glass doors opening into it, and a large window opening towards the river. On the ledge of the writing table is a large crucifix, an image of the Blessed Virgin, and four vases (two large and two small) of imitation flowers. On the table itself stood writing-desk, &c., check-books for linen, and a few religious books; a few pictures were hung round the room, including photographs of her confessor and friends. There were three chairs, a foot-stool, a small stove, and "fountain" for washing her hands.

The window had a Venetian blind outside.

There is a room for the women and *garçons* to damp the linen, and to wash their hands.

Over the linenry is a large room called the *"chambre de travail,"* or work-room. This has a superintending sister, two women, and a tailor, to examine and repair the cloth things for *employés* or patients.

The sister also has entire charge of all dry stores for the hospital use, and weighs and gives out the same to each sister according to her demand or *"bon,"* sewing silk, pins, needles, gutta-percha, &c.

This *"bon"* must in all cases be signed by the director and steward of the hospital.

A FRENCH "CHAMBRE DE LINGE À PANSEMENT," OR ROOM FOR THE LINEN REQUIRED FOR "DRESSINGS."

The *chambre de linge à pansement* consists of two small rooms on the upper floor for bandages, rollers, compresses, &c., and has a superintending sister, one woman, and an assistant sister. It is very much on the principle of the linenry; but here bandages, compresses, and the like, are only given once a week instead of every day.

Every Monday all bandages, compresses, &c., are written out and sent to La Pitié for the wash. They are returned in a week, but neither ironed nor mangled.

After they have been counted over, and compared with the list sent with them, the *mère* and assistants pare the edges, damp and fold or wind them, joining the smaller pieces together, and putting them by in tens or twenties.

The wards are supplied every week according to their demand, the applications for the same being entered in a book, and examined by the director and steward every quarter.

All bandages are numbered, and each number indicates a certain number of metres in length and inches in width varying from 6 m. to 14 m. or more.

On the first Monday in each month, the *mère* or sister superintendent writes out a list of the things she requires for "store," i. e., compresses of various sizes, bandages, linen slings for arms, &c. This "*bon*" is sent to the Salpêtrière, and she receives at once her demand in full.

She must enter in a book everything she receives, or gives out; adding the things in hand, to make her "count right."

Nevertheless, there are a certain number of bandages, compresses, and the like, which are too much worn to be of further use. These are used for any purpose into which they will cut; or, if utterly worn out, they are put by to send to the Salpêtrière, where they are made into "charpie."

All surgical bandages for the wards are made of linen, which is found in the end to be more economical than calico.

Medical and gum bandages are made of unbleached calico. These, when washed, are sent to the Central Bureau, for out-door patients.

Compresses are squares of linen which it is forbidden to cut or tear, as they are prepared of definite sizes.

All bandages and ordinary linings of splints are made in the Salpêtrière, and kept ready and prepared for use in the "Chambre de linge à pansement."

The above is an account of the *Lingerie* and *Chambre de linge à Pansement* , in the old Hotel-Dieu Hospital at Paris—where I worked for some months in 1869, under the Augustinian Sisters.

SECTION VII.

WARD DUTIES.

A sister, after seeing that the beds are properly made and aired, and giving out fresh sheets and draw sheets where required, and noticing that the wards are properly ventilated, should pay careful attention to seeing that all nuisances are removed, and the wards, closets, and lavatory swept and dry-rubbed, if of stained or oak flooring. With ordinary flooring, it is usual to have "scrubbers," who scrub the floors of the ward on alternate days.

The sister must take especial care that urinal bottles are washed with warm water and soda every morning, and kept bright and clean.

I would especially recommend their being made of clear glass without handles, but of the ordinary size and shape.

A moment's glance in walking down the wards, would show a sister or superintendent whether glass urinal bottles had been emptied as soon as used, and properly cleansed afterwards.

In preserving urine for the physician or surgeon, 1st, measure the quantity passed at the time; 2nd, fill one or more test tubes (according to order) with the same, and cover it with strapping, tightly fastened down; then gum or attach a small label with name and number of patient, and quantity passed.

Every patient ought to have a locker without sides, or double table. On the lower shelf should stand the urinal bottle, a spittoon with handle (of glass or white earthenware), brush and comb, soap in soap-dish, and shoes or slippers; the top shelf should hold a small hand-bell, a glass tumbler for drinking, a small white pot with lid, to contain milk or whatever may be allowed for drink during the day, a smaller pot with lid for butter, and a small tray for preserves or any other luxuries which his friends may bring, and which the patient may be permitted to have.

By being thus exposed to the light and air, the horrible fustiness of the hospital "locker" is avoided, and the sister is able to see at a glance whether the patient has any unwholesome or forbidden dainty or spirits; this she cannot do with the present system of closed lockers, for the patient always secretes such things in his bed, when the lockers are "turned out" for scrubbing.

At the head of each bedstead there should be a moveable stand for clothes, *i. e.*, a straight piece of wood, half-an-inch thick, about six feet high and two inches wide, placed on a firm pedestal. At the back of this should be placed hooks for the dressing-gown, and other articles of clothing, and a coloured calico or chintz bag for under linen.

The front of the stand should have a card bearing name of patient, disease, diet, and medicine.

A small linen bag for handkerchiefs should be attached to the head of the bedstead.

At King's College Hospital the clothes of the patients are kept in a large moveable box under each bed; this prevents the free current of air under the mattress, which is so desirable.

At University College Hospital (when I last visited it), the patient's clothes were placed under the mattress 'of the bed on which he lay; thus rendering the bed foul, and preventing the clothes from ever becoming sweet. I have since learnt, however, that they have adopted the same custom as at King's College Hospital.

At the Radcliffe Infirmary, Oxford, in the entrance corridor to the new ward, there are large cupboards for the clothes of the patients, and one for their hats and boots, with a separate drawer, numbered in correspondence with each bed.

It is also worthy of note, that the space under each bed in this Infirmary is covered with white glazed nonabsorbent tiles, so that no slop or dirt can either adhere or stain; and that there is a "sofa-table" for each patient. These tables (introduced by Dr. Acland) are the most practical I have seen, as they form also a chair and locker. The foot of each table being a small box or locker, raised from the floor by castors, makes a good seat, the back of which is formed by a simple but ingenious contrivance of the table itself.

The ordinary chamber utensil ought, properly speaking, to find no place in a well-regulated ward; but where these are used they should he of white glazed earthenware, with a well-fitting lid of the same material.

Bed-pans or bed-slippers should always be of glazed earthenware, not of metal, and with a well-fitting lid of the same material.

The edges of bed-pans should be greased or oiled. For ovariotomy and operation cases they should be warmed by being rinsed with warm water.

Bed-pans and chamber utensils are usually placed in the compartment where the water-closet is, or else in the lavatory. They should have special shelves, and only be taken into the ward when required. A label on each shelf should show how many that shelf contains.

A special cloth or towel should be hung in the same compartment to dry them with, when washed or warmed.

Whatever passes from a patient should be at once removed, and the vessel itself rinsed with cold water before being restored to its place.

As soon as the bed-pan has been used, and withdrawn from the patient, the lid should be immediately put on, the vessel emptied into the ward sink, and the water from the cock allowed to sweep through it.

Into the ward-sink should be poured all ward slops, the contents of chamber-pots, bed urinals, expectoration cups, wash-hand basins which have been used by bed-ridden patients, and the washings of wounds and sores: the utensils named should always be carefully cleansed with water from the watercock.

The sister must take especial care that these sinks, as well as the vessels kept in this compartment, are kept scrupulously clean.

Once or twice during the day, the sister must visit the water-closets of her ward to see that the pans and seats are kept perfectly clean and in working condition, and are free from smell.

Great care should be taken about the ventilation of the closets, and the door opening into the ward should be kept always shut.

There should be one towel to each patient, hung on two pegs in the lavatory: a third peg underneath should be for the brush and comb bag, unless there is a stand for it at the side, or head of the bed.

No patient should be permitted to use the towel of any other patient.

Those patients who are able to rise and dress, are expected to wash themselves in the stationary basins placed in the lavatory for that purpose.

Nothing should ever be thrown down the traps of these basins.

The sister must see, that the nurse whose duty it is, rinses and wipes carefully all basins and glasses that have been used; that the soap is dried, and everything put in order; and that all slops, on floor or woodwork, have been wiped up, before the lavatory is swept.

Wash-hand basins should be kept in the lavatory on a special shelf, and should be used solely for ordinary cleansing purposes, and on no account for any other.

The sister must see that these basins are half-filled with warm water, and carried to helpless patients in their beds, with the towel appropriated to their use, and that the nurses wash carefully such as are unable to wash themselves.

Where it is possible and allowed by the medical authority, all patients should on arrival have a bath before being put into bed.

Where this is not possible, the sister must have a mackintosh sheet placed entirely over the bed, and screens placed round it. The patient should then be covered with a blanket, and washed from head to foot, only a part being uncovered at a time, *i. e.*, first a foot and leg, and then when that is washed and dried, the other, and so on.

The waterproof sheeting having been withdrawn, a warm night-dress should be put on.

A draw-sheet should be put over the shoulders, and the hair combed by the nurse, who should hold a well-planed board close to the head, to prevent lice, if there are any, being combed into the bed; a result not uncommon.

Should the hair be much infested with lice, an order must be obtained from the house surgeon to have it cut short, and if necessary, a mixture must be rubbed in to destroy nits.

Twice a week, in the afternoon, when the work is slacker, the sister should see that those confined to their bed have their feet washed. The bed-clothes should be lifted at the foot of the bed, and a piece of mackintosh placed under the feet to prevent the mattress or sheet being wetted or soiled.

The feet should be washed, one at a time, with a piece of flannel kept for that purpose, and warm soap and water, and dried with a soft towel.

All patients, who can do so, should have a warm bath once a week.

After the bedmaking and the washing, sister will see that the nurses pay proper attention to the prevention of bed-sores, in cases where long confinement to bed has happened, or is likely to happen; especially where evacuations are passed involuntarily; in these the greatest attention to cleanliness is demanded.

Every morning, a screen having been placed round the bed, the patient's back or side on which he lies should be thoroughly washed with soap and warm water, and dried afterwards with a soft towel.

A little "violet" powder or oxide of zinc may be used to ensure perfect dryness to the skin. In hospitals where I have worked, I have found the following used, the skin having been first carefully washed and dried.

> At King's College Hospital, collodion (gun cotton dissolved in ether), painted on in one brushful, without break.
> At St. Thomas's Hospital, the skin was rubbed with brandy or rectified spirit.
> In Germany, as at St. Thomas's: lemons cut in half are also used; the back, after being washed, is rubbed with the juice.
> In France, an ointment composed of two drachms of tannate of lead, and one ounce of cerate, is used.

Where the surgeons prefer spreading the dressings themselves, or where there are no ledges to the beds, two stools about the height of small tables should be placed in the centre at the two ends of the ward. They should be covered with mackintosh, and everything put on them that will be required, ointments, lotions, bandages, lint, tow, cotton wool, strapping, pins, sponges, linen compresses, and a clean draw-sheet.

By the side should stand two earthenware buckets, highly glazed, and with lids; one should be for dirty water, the other for soiled dressings; there should also be two cans for water, hot and cold; a tin "strapping cup" for heating the plaister; and a basket with lid for soiled bandages.

Small shallow vessels of various sizes are required to receive discharges, or to hold lotions.

When these buckets are full, they must be carried at once into the compartment of the ward sink, and emptied into the sink, or thrown down the shoot intended for that purpose.

Should it not be permitted to pass soiled dressings or poultices down the sink, they should be kept in the glazed earthenware bucket with lid in the water-closet compartment, until the scrubber can take them downstairs to the ash-hole or place appointed to receive them.

The sister should see that the dressings are ready before the patient's wound is uncovered.

The poultices should be made in the ward scullery on a board for that purpose; and each nurse should leave everything she has used in perfect order and cleanliness after the dressings are completed.

A sister should never allow a linseed meal poultice to be made before the wound has been properly washed and cared for; this being done, it should be lightly covered with a piece of linen, wet or dry, and the poultice made and applied.

The sister should personally inspect all wounds before they are dressed by the nurse.

In special cases, where she dreads carelessness or forgetfulness on the part of a nurse, it is necessary to inspect also when the dressing is over.

A nurse who is habitually careless or forgetful should be dismissed.

The sister must daily examine the baths, which are usually in the lavatory, and observe whether they have been properly cleansed and dried.

In going over a ward of one of our London hospitals some little time ago I asked to see one of the baths; the cover was removed, and the whole bath was seen to be filled with dust, cobwebs, and "creeping things;" the sister in some confusion said that "it had not been used for some time," and was absolutely ignorant whether the taps were or were not in working order.

Apart from the fact that there should be no covered recesses for dust or cobwebs in or near a ward, imagine the consequences if the bath were wanted on a sudden for a patient, and it was found that the taps were useless or refused to act!

The floors should be swept after every meal, and after the "dressings."

Sweeping should be effectual, but should be managed in such a manner as not to fill the atmosphere with dust. The broom should not be used recklessly, but should be carried gently and steadily over the floor, bearing the dust before it. Where there is much dust, the floor may be sprinkled before being swept, with wet tea-leaves when obtainable, or the broom may be dipped lightly into water. The dirt should be carried away in dust pans.

Scrubbing is to be resorted to whenever necessary to effect cleanliness. Sand is better than soap for scrubbing well-made floors.

The reckless use of water is to be avoided. It soaks through the cracks of the floor into apartments below, if there are any, and leaves dampness behind.

Not merely the floors, but the walls, windows, and painted woodwork, require to be kept scrupulously clean.

The walls should be dusted from time to time, and kept free from dirt and cobwebs.

Windows should be washed once a week. Here, as in scrubbing, a caution may be given against the excessive use of water.

Ordinary deal flooring should not be washed or wetted more than once in the day, but merely swept after meals and dressings, for the wood is too porous, and the moisture it absorbs, set free afterwards by evaporation, vitiates the atmosphere for the patients.

Where floors are of oak, it is usual to polish them immediately after the doctor's visit with bees'-wax fastened to a pole, and a hard brush attached to the sole of the foot by small straps. The floor should then be "dry-rubbed," *i.e.*, a two-foot square of flannel, about two or three thicknesses, is placed loose under the foot, and gently pushed up and down over the floor.

In the case of anything being spilt upon the floor, it should be at once wiped up, and the surface sponged, cleaned, and brushed.

Every three months the floor should be thoroughly *washed* with soft soap and hot water. When dry, it should be "wiped over" with a mixture of melted bees'-wax, and sufficient hard yellow soap, cut down and dissolved in it, to make the wax work smoothly. When this is dry, the whole flooring should be thoroughly polished with brushes on the feet.

This was the method observed in the chief military hospital of France, the Val-de-Grâce; and by a little extra exertion on the part of the sister, and by the preparation of some special little treat for those who had this "extra cleaning," it was regarded rather as a pleasure than otherwise.

Where the floors are painted, or stained, the sister must have a damp cloth passed under all the beds, and over the whole ward, at least twice in the day, the whole being afterwards carefully dried with a dry flannel.

In Germany they clean the painted floors this way. They are first swept with an ordinary soft-haired broom. Then a bucket of water, another broom of short hard hair, and a very coarse linen floor-cloth are brought. The floor-cloth is dipped in the bucket, and fitted, "wringing wet" (as servants would say), over the broom, which is then passed rapidly up and down under the beds and along the floor, like an ordinary mop; the floor-cloth is dipped again in the bucket, washed out, and wrung dry. It is again placed on the broom, and the rubbing up and down resumed until the boards look dry.

This is done throughout the whole ward the first thing in the morning, and after meals; for although in the latter case the floors are swept, and wiped over with a damp cloth, neither so much water nor so much time is devoted to them as in the first great cleaning.

Stoves and fireplaces must be kept well blacked, and the ashes must be removed the first thing in the morning and afterwards during the day as often as necessary, with as little dust as possible.

Gas-burners should be cleaned once a week.

The latrines require careful attention, and their supervision in male wards is an important part of the duties of the sister of the ward.

All lockers should be highly polished. If of oak, they should be cleaned just as the oak flooring is cleaned, with the difference of being polished and rubbed by hand.

They should be dusted after each meal.

If of stained or polished wood, a damp cloth should be passed over them, after the floor has been swept, and this should be done after every meal.

Every article placed on them should be kept clean and bright.

Each patient should, if possible, have a chair by his bed.

There should be at least two easy-chairs in each ward.

Chairs should be merely dusted.

Linen shoots are intended for passing at once into the foul linen closet in the basement all changes or soiled articles of ward linen, such as sheets, pillow-cases, shirts, nightdresses, bandages, and similar articles.

The articles should be done up in parcels small enough to pass readily down the shoot without any force being used. They should be so wrapped up as not to soil the tube in passing. Nothing but foul linen and dressings should be passed down the shoots.

The shoots should be examined from time to time, to see that they are in good order, and clean inside.

Each quantity of foul linen should be accompanied by a check or list, showing the number and description of articles, and the ward to which they belong. They must be counted out by one of the nurses before the sister of the ward, who should write down the number of each article as it was named, and sign it with her name and the date.

In all English hospitals it is usual to change the linen at least twice in the week; in some hospitals this is done four times. In French hospitals it is changed five times, the two days excepted being Wednesday, when the clean clothes come back from the wash, and Sunday, when all extra work is avoided as much as possible.

The rule in all hospitals, English and foreign, is that the sister should receive from the linen room the same number and description of clean linen articles, as of soiled ones sent by her down the foul linen shoot.

The linen arrangements in the French hospitals are said to be the best in the world; and therefore I have devoted a section to the "Lingerie," containing the notes made on the French system during the time that I was undergoing my "training" with the Roman Catholic sisters in Paris.

Every sister has a certain amount of linen in store in her ward. She has to keep an accurate account of this, and of the quantity in use.

It is usual to give an inventory of the linen and medical comforts, if any, to the sister of the ward upon her first taking charge of it; but where this is not done, the sister's first duty must be to make one for herself, with the aid of one of her nurses. This she can afterwards get the matron or superintendent to verify.

It should be neatly written out, and signed with her name, the ward, and the date.

In all good modern hospitals, there is a kitchen or scullery attached to the ward, for washing up cups and saucers, plates, spoons, and other small articles of ward equipment connected with the dieting of the sick. This room being also used as a day-room by the nurses of the ward, it is sometimes difficult to keep it in that perfect order which is desirable.

I recommend, therefore, to sisters of wards a plan which I adopted myself with great success. Having found remonstrances useless in preventing nurses from putting caps, aprons, and other articles into cupboards and places where they had no business to be, and having found that the excuse always was that the things had just been "laid down for a moment," I informed nurses and probationers that such things would always be removed by myself, and that therefore, if they lost anything, they might come to me for it.

SECTION VIII.

BEDDING AND BED-MAKING.

At whatever hour a sister may enter her wards, whether at 5 a.m. or 7 a.m., she is to be present at the bed-making, and should be in the ward before the day nurses and probationers, that she may "check off" each name in her note-book as they appear.

This rule should be observed during the day at all hours, when nurses and probationers come on duty. She should then, after receiving the report of the night nurses, visit each of the patients, and make notes of any cases to which the doctor's attention is to be specially called, on account of disagreement with the night nurses' report, or from other causes.

The chief thing to attend to in making a bed is to arrange it as smoothly as possible, and to keep the bedclothes under and over the patient free from wrinkles.

When there is any tendency to bed-sore, a blanket should never be placed under the patient. To use Miss Nightingale's words, "It retains damp, and acts like a poultice." In cold weather, however, medical men in England sometimes order it for their patients; but it is never used in the best hospitals abroad, and it certainly adds to the difficulty of keeping the bed smooth.

In the French civil hospitals, and in some few wards in English hospitals, iron bedsteads with "rheochne springs" are used; these are permeable by the air up to the very mattress.

These bedsteads the Sœurs Augustines, at the Hôtel Dieu, always brushed and cleansed thoroughly, or saw cleansed, once a week in medical, and once a fortnight in surgical wards; the patient being moved bodily, mattress and all, to a temporary bed, whilst this cleansing process was carried on. I wish that these iron spring bedsteads could be introduced into our hospitals.

In England the ordinary iron bedstead is used, but unless a patient dies, or has suffered from some contagious disease, a cleansing process is never considered necessary; a fact which, I think, partly accounts for the vermin which are the curse and disgrace of some of our good hospitals, and which in foreign hospitals are almost unknown.

The best bed is a horse-hair mattress, but it is a great mistake to place a cotton or straw mattress beneath.

Over the mattress a clean sheet should be evenly placed, the sides and ends being well tucked in under the mattress, so as to prevent the sheet from being wrinkled, when the patient moves in bed; sufficient should be left at the top to allow of its being drawn under and then over the bolster from the back; in fact, to allow of the bolster being rolled in it.

The pillow should be enclosed in a separate case.

The upper bedclothes should consist of a sheet, and one or more blankets, according to the weather; these should be carefully tucked in.

Dark-coloured or heavy quilts should never be used, the "virtue" of the former, their not showing the dirt, being in fact a great drawback.

You should never use anything for the sick or wounded which is dirty, or which does not show the dirt.

At the Val-de-Grâce in Paris, and in the Crown Princess's "Ambulance," nothing but blankets were used as coverlets, and the general effect was bright and good.

In the civil French hospitals, it is customary, however, to use a sheet as a quilt, and this for many reasons is preferable to any mode with which I am acquainted, as a sheet can be washed more frequently than a blanket, and at less cost.

This sheet is put on first; that is to say, the two corners of the bottom of the sheet are pulled through the iron bars, or sacking, of the bedstead, and pinned with large safety-pins. The mattress is then put on, and the bed made, and when it is well tucked in all round, the sheet-quilt is pulled up over all, and left free.

In surgical wards, in beds for knee diseases and the like, this quilt should not be pinned under the mattress, but, as well as the blankets, should be folded back at the foot, ready to be turned up at a moment's notice.

This sheet is used afterwards, in French hospitals, as a top-sheet for the patient, his top-sheet being taken for the under-sheet.

Sheets are changed twice a week, as in English hospitals, i.e., one clean sheet is put on the bed on Sunday, and another on Thursday, the clean being always employed as the quilt. They are of course changed oftener if required, and if soiled are entirely removed.

Draw-sheets in French hospitals are always changed five times in twenty-four hours, viz., thrice during the day, and twice during the night.

Draw-sheets should always be much smaller in every respect than ordinary ones, and the latter should never, on any consideration, be allowed to be used in their stead.

Changing the under-sheet without moving the patient, as after operations, is a matter of some difficulty, and a nurse usually requires the aid of one or more assistants.

The nurse first loosely rolls the clean sheet, which should not only be well aired, but warmed, leaving sufficient to cover the bolster. The soiled sheets must be unrolled from the bolster while the clean one is arranged in its place; the two sheets are then drawn down together.

Where the patient can be turned on his side, much fatigue may be saved him, by changing the sheet in the same manner as a draw-sheet is changed, viz., roll up half the clean sheet lengthwise, then loosen the soiled sheet, and press it up closely against the back of the patient; arrange the clean sheet evenly in the vacant space, with the rolled part resting against the soiled roll, and pressed tightly into the back. The patient should now be gently rolled or lifted on to the clean side of the bed, the soiled sheet immediately withdrawn, and the clean one unrolled in its place.

It is needless to add that in severe fever and in other cases attended by unconsciousness, the soiled draw-sheet should be first folded under the patient, who must then be carefully cleansed, before it is rolled, or the clean one put in its place.

A piece of waterproof, about 3 feet or 3½ feet square, is desirable as a protection for the mattress and under-sheet from getting wet or soiled, but it should not be used instead of a draw-sheet, as it is unpleasant for the patient to have it next him, except in operation cases, abscesses, or any cases where there is much discharge, such as diarrhœa, dysentery, hernia, lithotomy, ovariotomy, hæmorrhage, or the like.

It was usual in German hospitals to tie this waterproof sheeting by tapes to the side of the bedstead, and pin or tie the draw-sheet over it.

The sister of the ward should always see that her "severe cases" receive stimulant, if the patient is taking any, or nourishment of some kind, immediately before or after his sheets are changed, as the process is often exhausting to a patient.

A patient should never be told that his bed is to be "changed," as nurses term it, till everything is ready, and it should then be done as quietly and rapidly as possible. And let a nurse remember it is a chief part of good nursing that the beds of her patients, as well as her patients themselves, should always look, as well as be, clean.

SECTION IX.

ADMINISTRATION OF MEDICINES, SUPPOSITORIES, AND ENEMATA; INSTRUCTION CONCERNING HYPODERMIC INJECTIONS AND PASSING THE CATHETER.

It is usually the duty of the ward-sister herself to administer the medicines, but sometimes she has simply to see that the nurses administer it at the appointed hours. In the performance of this duty a nurse cannot be too punctual or too precise.

It will be her duty, therefore, to see that the nurse has at such times, in addition to a measuring glass, a small basin of clear water and a glass cloth, as the medicine glass after having been used for one patient should be rinsed and wiped, before being used for another. A separate measure should be kept for oily or strong-smelling medicines.

When medicines are volatile they ought to be swallowed the instant they are poured into the glass. The bottle should be immediately corked.

When medicines are to be given in a state of effervescence the dose of the medicine should be poured upon that of the lemon juice previously put into a tumbler.

Powders should be mixed with pounded white sugar and a little water or milk; or with moist sugar, or with treacle.

The nauseous taste of castor oil is covered by warm milk, or by coffee. It is much diminished when the oil is floated upon cold water, and a teaspoonful of brandy floated upon the oil.

In France, it is given in a warm "soupe maigre" (vegetable soup), which is the most palatable form I know. In Germany it is given to children in moist brown sugar.

If a patient be unable to take pills the pill should be put into a morsel of soft bread, or into a mass of any conserve and washed down. The smaller the pills the greater is the difficulty of swallowing them.

In France it is usual for the sister to put a small piece of damped rice paper into a table-spoon, and then fold it round the pill, or pills. The spoon is then filled with water, and placed by the sister well back in the throat of the patient, who swallows the mass without difficulty.

The saline purgative known as "Epsom salts" should be administered in a quantity of water only sufficient for its solution; and a large basin of warm gruel or weak tea should be given an hour afterwards.

"Suppositories" are medicines in a solid form, introduced into the rectum or vagina, generally either to relieve pain, or to act as astringents.

When the patients cannot apply the remedy, they should be directed to lie on the left side, with the knees drawn up, and to make an effort to bear down. The sister or nurse standing behind, should at the same moment pass her hand under the sheet and introduce the suppository into the anus.

ENEMATA.

Injections into the bowel are called by this name.

They may be either medicinal or nutritive.

The patient should be directed to lie on the left side with the knees drawn up where this is possible.

The tube of the enema apparatus should be well oiled, and the sister or nurse standing at the back of the patient should pass her hand under the sheet, and introduce it not more than four inches into the anal orifice upward and backward, holding it steadily there while the syringe is worked.

When purgative enemata are used, the fluid should be injected gently and gradually; and immediately after the prescribed quantity has been thrown into the bowel, and the tube withdrawn, a towel folded into a ball should be pressed against the fundament so as to favour the retention of the enema for some minutes.

On no account whatever should any force be used in introducing the tube or mouthpiece of the syringe into the rectum.

The injection should be stopped at once on the patient saying that he cannot bear any more.

The fluids usually injected into the bowel are—

Warm water, alone or, with sufficient soap rubbed down into it, to render it creamy. From a few ounces to a pint of warm water, with one ounce of soft soap, is often effectual when it is not desired to act strongly on the bowels.

Half an ounce or an ounce of castor oil, a dessert or table-spoonful of common salt, Epsom salts and senna, or turpentine, added to a few ounces or a pint of warm water or thin gruel, form the purgative enemata most generally used.

Laudanum, added to two ounces of thin starch or arrow-root, is the sedative injection generally employed. The quantity used is directed by the doctor, according to the age of the patient, and other circumstances. The starch or arrow-root should be made with cold water.

Nutritive enemata should be always small; for the smaller their bulk the more likely they are to be retained. They should never exceed four ounces of fluid.

They should be very slowly injected, so as not to stimulate the bowel to reject them.

They may consist of beef tea, soup, milk, or milk and eggs beaten up together, thickened with arrow-root or corn-flour.

If it be advisable to combine stimulant action with the nutritive, brandy may be added in such dose as the physician directs.

HYPODERMIC INJECTIONS.

Of late years the method of giving anodynes by hypodermic injections has been largely employed. It is usual now after operations. The quantity used is small, and the solutions are very powerful. One grain of morphia in six minims is a common strength, and two minims a common dose. In introducing the needle, a fold of the skin is to be taken up between the finger and thumb, and with the other hand the needle is to be firmly passed horizontally to the depth of about half an inch.

Then the two minims are to be slowly introduced by turning the screw of the instrument twice, or by pressing the piston gently till the marks show that the quantity has entered.

PASSING THE CATHETER.

The sister or nurse is occasionally called upon to relieve an attack of retention of urine in females and children, by the introduction of a short catheter, to draw the water off. This should be done without exposing the patient.

For females the simplest plan is to make the patient lie upon her back, with the thighs separated and slightly drawn up. The sister or nurse having oiled the second finger of her right hand, should then introduce it between the labia, close to the arch of the pubis, with the palm of the hand upwards; along the finger, as on a director, she slips the instrument (previously well oiled) held lightly in the left hand. Thus the catheter cannot enter the vagina, while it will almost certainly slip into the orifice of the urethra.

It will easily slip into the bladder, provided there be no obstruction. This may be known by feeling its point move freely in a cavity, and by the urine flowing through it.

For male children the catheter having been warmed, well oiled, and being held loosely in the right hand, should be introduced into the orifice of the urethra, (the handle being directed to one or other side,) and passed gently along the canal. Meanwhile the organ must be held with the left hand and gently drawn above the catheter in moderate tension. When the point of the catheter has reached the membranous part of the urethra its handle should be brought into the middle line and kept there; then, by depressing the point of the instrument and drawing the handle away from the abdomen, still keeping accurately in the middle line, the instrument will usually easily slip into the bladder, provided there be no obstruction.

The point of the catheter often stops when it has reached the membranous part of the urethra, and if the depression of the point does not cause it to pass on, it should be withdrawn for a short distance, and again glided on in the same manner.

If this does not succeed, the forefinger of the left hand, having been oiled or greased, should be introduced into the rectum, and its palmar surface brought in contact with the convexity of the catheter. Then, by raising this part of the instrument, and at the same time gently pushing it forwards, it will in most cases be tilted into the bladder. This may be known by feeling its point move freely in a cavity, and by the urine flowing through it.

When a catheter is to be removed from the bladder, its handle should be laid hold of and drawn back towards the abdomen, the instrument at the same time being lifted from the urethra. The point of the finger should be pressed on the orifice, to prevent any fluid escaping from it during its removal.

It is sometimes necessary to wash out the bladder or inject fluids into it; for this purpose a full-sized catheter is required, and a large syringe or India-rubber bag fitted with a nozzle and stop-cock. Great gentleness should be used, especial care being taken to steady the catheter when working the syringe, so that its extremity will not be forced against the walls of the bladder.

It should be remembered that in elderly women who have had children, as well as in pregnant females, the meatus is often drawn into the vagina, somewhat under the symphysis pubis.

SECTION X.

DRY HEAT, MOIST HEAT, INHALATION, AND THE USE OF SPRAY DISPERSER.

To raise the temperature of certain parts of the body, and to relieve pain, dry heat is often ordered. It may be applied by means of hot flannels, tins, or bottles filled with hot water, by dry heated bricks, and by bags of heated sand, or bran.

Flannel being of a loose texture, and involving air, is a bad conductor of heat; when heated it should be put together as loosely as possible, and applied in that state to the skin. It should never be covered by a towel, or linen, as that augments its radiating property. White flannel retains heat much longer than black, or any coloured flannel.

Stomach plates and other solid media for applying warmth to the body should be covered with white or coloured flannel, according as they may be required to communicate an immediate or intense heat, or to convey a slighter but more permanent stimulus to the part requiring to be heated.

To apply dry heat to the surface of the body generally, the hot air, or lamp bath, is bath, is used. The temperature may be raised from 100° to 160°, according to the requirements of the case.

The patient must have his clothes removed, and a blanket thrown over him; he should then be covered, while in bed, by a bamboo frame about 5 feet long, 18 inches high, and 2 feet wide, the end being arranged so as to fit close round the neck.

The frame must be covered over with blankets sufficient to retain the heated air; and the blanket covering the patient under the framework be removed.

A small covered vessel containing burning charcoal may then be placed inside the frame, near the foot; or the air may be heated by means of a lamp placed under a trumpet-shaped tube communicating with the interior of the frame. In the Turkish bath the air of the whole room is heated and the person breathes the heated air.

The hot air, or lamp bath, should last about 20 minutes.

MOIST HEAT.

Either the whole or only a part of the body may be immersed. When the former is required, the bath should be large enough to immerse the whole of the body as high as the neck.

A thermometer should always be used to see the exact temperature.

Whatever description of bath is ordered to be used, the same temperature must be maintained the whole time that the patient remains in the bath. At the end of 10 or 15 minutes the water should be tested by a thermometer and more hot water added if necessary.

The medium period for remaining in the bath is from 10 to 15 minutes, unless otherwise ordered by the medical man.

After getting out of the bath the patient must be quickly dried by a warm sheet being thrown over him, and the body rapidly shampooed; his night-dress being then put on, be should be sent to bed.

Where a medicated bath has been ordered, a blanket should be thrown over the patient instead of a sheet upon his coming out of the bath: he should be sent immediately to bed, and covered up with extra blankets to encourage free perspiration, for an hour or so at least.

When he has become cool, he should be thoroughly dried, and his night-dress, well-warmed, put on as usual.

The quantity of water used for a hip bath should be only sufficient to fill a little more than one-third of the vessel employed.

The patient should be placed in a semi-reclining or sitting posture with the thighs well flexed.

If it is required to excite the womb to greater activity, when the monthly secretion is defective, the heat of the bath should be as high as it can be borne; but the time of remaining in it should not exceed 15 minutes.

When a full-sized bath cannot be had, a convenient and pleasant warm bath is made by laying a blanket in the hip bath. The patient then sitting down, the now warm and moist blanket is wrapped over him, next the skin, and another blanket is thrown over him and the bath.

A foot-bath should be large enough to receive both the feet placed side by side, and high enough to reach to the knees.

It should be three parts filled with water.

As a foot-bath is chiefly intended to cause derivation, it should be used as hot as it can be borne, and always hot enough to redden the skin of the part immersed.

	Water. Fahr.	Vapour. Fahr.	Air. Fahr.
Cold	33°—65°		
Cool	65°—75°		
Temperate	75°—85°		
Tepid	85°—92°	90°—100°	96°—106°
Warm	92°—98°	100°—115°	106°—120°
Hot	98°—112°	115°—140°	120°—180°

Fomentations may be regarded as local bathing, the intention being to convey heat combined with moisture.

Coarse flannel cloths, with the ends sewn together, wrung out of boiling water, by means of two sticks turned in opposite directions, form the best fomentations.

They should be shaken up, and laid lightly over the part, and covered with mackintosh, or oiled silk.

Ordinary fomenting flannels should be about three yards long; any coarse flannel, however, soaked in boiling water and wrung out by placing it in a towel or cloth, and by twisting it in opposite directions, may be used for the purpose.

If counter-irritation is desired, the cloth is sprinkled with one to two tablespoonfuls of turpentine immediately before its application.

It should be changed every 10 minutes or quarter of an hour, and then be immediately replaced by another soaked flannel, which has been made ready while the first was being removed.

Spongio-piline is a good material for fomentation.

A double layer of lint, wrung in a towel after being steeped in boiling water, and covered with light india-rubber cloth, forms the best fomentation for long-continued application.

The fluids used for fomenting are of various kinds, such as poppy water, mallow water; and camomile-flower water.

For poppy water take 4 oz. of dried poppyheads; break them to pieces, and empty out the seeds. Then boil the shells in 3 or down to 2 pints of water for a quarter of an hour. Strain through a cloth or sieve, and keep the water for use.

For mallow-water, take 4 oz. of dried mallows, and boil in 4 pints of water for a quarter a of an hoar, and strain.

Sometimes 2 oz. of camomile flowers are boiled with either of these.

The method of applying heat and moisture in affections of the throat and chest is termed inhalation. An apparatus called an "inhaler" is found in all hospitals. In pouring the boiling water into the inhaler, it should be remembered that it should be only half filled, so as to allow ample space for steam and air.

The patient should place the mouthpiece in, or against the mouth, and breathe quietly.

An ingenious apparatus has been contrived for the formation of spray, and for its inhalation. The usual form of it is that of two india-rubber balls, by which air is forced so rapidly through a tube as to cause a vacuum in a lower tube below it, and the rapid rise of liquid from the bottle in which the tube is fixed.

This instrument supplies the place of gargles, and is a great comfort to patients who have sore mouths, quinsy, or sordes.

Iced water, or medicated substances, such as carbolic acid and glycerine, are thus used.

SECTION XI.

POULTICES: APPLICATION OF COLD, AND USE OF SIPHONS.

Poultices are employed in the treatment of abscesses, suppurating wounds, inflammation, and pain.

"Scald out a basin, for you can never make a good poultice unless you have perfectly boiling water," said Abernethy. Then pour in boiling water according to the size of the poultice required, adding gradually sufficient linseed-meal for a linseed-meal poultice to form a thick paste, stirring thoroughly the whole time one way until it is of the proper consistence and smoothness.

It should be spread on linen or tow, according to the usage in the hospital, the edge in both cases being doubled back on itself, and then folded over the edge of the poultice, or "tucked" in, as nurses say.

If the spatula, with which the poultice is made, be dipped into hot water while spreading it, it will spread more smoothly.

A little simple dressing or olive oil may be added where a poultice is to remain undisturbed for many hours.

Oil-silk, oiled paper, or mackintosh should always be placed over linseed-meal poultices; like fomentations, they are intended to convey heat with moisture.

For a bread poultice scald out a basin; then, having put in some hot water, throw in coarsely crumbled bread, and stir briskly. Cover it with a plate, and put it by the fire to soak for about 5 minutes. Spread and apply it in the ordinary way.

If this is to be used as an evaporating poultice, it should not be covered with oil-silk.

A bread and milk poultice is made in precisely the same way, using boiling milk instead of water.

An astringent poultice is made by mixing a drachm of powdered alum with the white of two eggs.

For a carbon poultice take 2 ounces of bread crumb, and soak for 10 minutes in 10 oz. of boiling water; then mix and add gradually ½oz. wood charcoal, 1½ oz. linseed-meal. The whole should be well stirred together, and then spread and applied in the ordinary manner.

The quantity of the articles may be increased or diminished, according to the size of the poultice, but the proportion should be the same. Sometimes only a quarter of an ounce is mixed in the poultice, the other quarter ounce being sprinkled over the surface of the poultice when it is spread.

A chlorinated soda poultice is made like a linseed-meal poultice, but consists of two parts of linseed-meal to one of chlorinated soda, mixed with boiling water.

A sedative poultice is composed of hemlock leaf, one part; linseed-meal, three parts; and sufficient boiling water.

A yeast poultice is made by mixing a pound of flour or linseed-meal, or oatmeal, with half a pint of yeast or beer grounds.

The mixture is to be heated in a pot, carefully stirred, to prevent burning, and when sufficiently warm must be spread on linen like any other poultice.

For a carrot poultice boil carrots until soft; strain, and mix with bread or linseed-meal to the consistence of a poultice.

An anodyne poultice is made by mixing linseed-meal with decoction of poppies in lieu of simple boiling water, or by sprinkling a drachm of laudanum over an ordinary poultice.

For a mustard poultice mix equal parts of good mustard and linseed meal with sufficient boiling water to make a paste. It should be spread on two folds of linen rag, or on paper covered with muslin.

A very strong poultice may be made by mixing mustard and water alone, as above.

A mild stimulant poultice may be made by dusting a little mustard over an ordinary linseed-meal poultice.

APPLICATION OF COLD.

Cold may be used to arrest bleeding, or subdue inflammation.

The principal intention of many lotions is to abstract heat from inflamed surfaces by the evaporation which they produce.

The inflamed or hot part, therefore, should be covered with a single layer of thin linen or muslin—the thinner it is the better—and kept constantly cool by dropping cold water or an evaporating lotion on it.

The best way of keeping it wet is by means of a piece of worsted passing to it from a vessel raised somewhat above the part; or a small siphon may be fitted to the vessel, by which the amount of fluid can be accurately controlled.

The bed near the part must be arranged with mackintosh, raised on a small pad towards the centre, and with a broad piece hanging over the mattress at the side to carry off superfluous water. A tub of some sort should be put to receive it.

Ice should be broken up into pieces about an inch in size, and put into a bladder, or into an india-rubber ice-bag.

The bladder should not be more than half full, and it should be securely tied around the neck. If the head is to be kept cool, the bladder should be suspended by tape, so as just to reach the head. With a bent hair-pin, the tape can be easily shortened or lengthened. In other cases it should be attached to the cradle placed over the part where the application is required.

Dr. Stokes considers the best way of applying ice to the head is to place a smooth piece of ice two or three inches long and one and a half broad, in a cup of soft sponge, and pass it round and round over the head. The sponge absorbs the water, and the pain of the cold is avoided. When the sponge is saturated, it is to be squeezed, and the ice is to be replaced. The head should be shaved, or the hair cut close.

SECTION XII.

WARD DRESSINGS, AND REQUISITES FOR SAME.

As I have already said, a sister must never allow a wound to be uncovered until everything is at hand which will be required, and the dressing itself prepared.

The only exception being burns, and those wounds which require poulticing. These should have the old dressings removed, the discharges cleaned away from the edges of the wound and surrounding parts, before the poultice is made (unless a second nurse can be spared for this duty) and applied.

Where the nurse has to make the poultices herself, she should lightly cover the wound with a piece of clean linen until the poultice is ready.

In the case of a patient who is burnt over a large surface of the body, only a small part should be uncovered at a time.

The greatest care must be taken in removing dressings. If adherent to a wound, they should be moistened by bathing with warm water.

In removing dressings from wounds which contain ligatures or sutures it should be seen that the dressing is not sticking to them. If necessary, the ends of the stitches or ligatures may be cut across and removed with the dressing.

Tow soaked in water is better than sponges for cleaning the edges of a wound.

The surface of a wound is best cleaned by using an American india-rubber syringe, with a rose-top fitted to it, as by alternately making and relaxing pressure on the central ball a continuous flow of water may be maintained.

Nurses should always wash and dry their hands after dressing a wound.

They should be careful never to touch their eyes or lips whilst their hands are soiled from dressings.

If they have any crack or cut on their hands, they should cover it with strapping before commencing the dressings, and, when these are concluded, should wash their hands in water containing Condy's or other disinfecting fluid.

Every nurse—in addition to a large pair of scissors blunt at the points, and pocket pincushion hung at her side—should have a small pocket leather case, containing the following:—

1 pair dressing forceps.

1 pair sharp-pointed scissors.

1 razor, useful in shaving the hairy surface near a wound.

1 silver probe, with eye at one end.

1 silver probe, with a short flattened handle.

1 penknife.

1 pencil and memorandum-card.

Needles, white thread, silk, and thimble.

1 spatula.

1 caustic-holder.

The French sisters always carried matches and a wax taper in their pockets, for emergencies. While I was being trained under them I did the same, and often found them most useful.

I have already mentioned, in the Section on Ward Duties, that everything required for the dressings must be placed in readiness before they are begun.

Dry lint or old soft linen may be used for dry dressings.

If to promote the union of a wound by first intention, take two pieces, an inch or two in width, and a little longer than the wound; apply one on each side of it, but not over it, and a third piece large enough to cover all.

They are retained *in situ* by a bandage or a strip or two of plaister.

Water-dressing is the application to a sore or wound of a piece of lint, soft linen, or charpie, soaked in water, and covered with oiled silk, gutta-percha, or, better still, thin india-rubber cloth.

The lint should be slightly larger than the wound, and the outer covering must overlap the lint all round.

A bandage will secure the dressing. In France and Germany a linen compress is put over the oiled silk or gutta-percha before the bandage is applied.

It needs to be changed twice or three times a day, and sometimes twice during the night.

The dressing may be prepared with warm or cold water, as the medical man shall direct.

The various kinds of lotions which are applied to sores or unhealthy surfaces are used in the same way as water-dressings, the lint or linen being soaked in the lotion instead of the water.

Greasy dressings are chiefly used for superficial sores, and in dressing a blistered surface. They consist of various ointments spread on linen, charpie, or lint.

The ointment ordered should be spread smoothly and evenly on the lint, and laid on the sore. It may be retained by a strip of adhesive plaister or by a bandage.

Adhesive plaister is used when it is desirable to keep the edges of a wound together, or to give support or to procure pressure.

The plaister is cut into strips, the width and length depending upon the size of the wound, or the nature of the part to be covered.

In dressing a simple incised wound, the strips should be narrow, and made to cross each other in the centre, the edges of the wound being first brought together by the finger and thumb. If it can be avoided, the entire surface of a wound should not be covered with the plaister, as it prevents the escape of discharge.

Great care should be taken in removing plaister from wounds, for if one end of the strip be laid hold of and drawn roughly away, it may very easily open out a wound, or destroy its adhesions. When necessary to remove it, one end must be drawn first gently towards the wound, and when the strip is loosened so far, the other end must be removed in the same way, and so on, strip by strip.

Bathing the plaister with warm water, and rubbing a little oil over it, will sometimes assist its removal.

The substance of which the plaister is composed often adheres to the skin and cannot be washed off. A little oil rubbed over it will remove it completely.

In bandaging a limb or joint with strapping, the plaister—cut into broad strips—is to be applied in such a way that each strip shall overlap the preceding one by about a third of its width.

Scott's dressing is merely the application of mercurial ointment (spread on strips of lint) to the surface of a joint, strips of plaister being then carried round it so as to embrace the entire articulation.

Strapping applied to the breast to support it, or exercise pressure upon it, should be cut not less than 24 inches in length, and about two inches in width, and then adjusted in the most convenient direction.

The art of bandaging, as has been implied in the account of the French Infirmiers, is a special art, requiring both instruction and practice.

SECTION XIII.

THE APPLICATION OF LEECHES; DIRECTIONS CONCERNING CUPPING AND BLISTERING.

When leeches are about to be applied to any part, it should first be well washed with a little soap and warm water; then with simple cold water; and lastly, it should be well dried.

If held in the hand or placed upon a dry towel, leeches will often refuse to bite, and various expedients are resorted to, in order to induce them to take hold, such as cold cream, a little milk, or fresh blood smeared upon the skin; but these will generally fail if the leeches have been ill treated or handled too much, and fresh ones must be procured.

If it is a flat surface, the leeches are best applied in the following manner:—Put them into a wine glass filled with water; cover it with a piece of paper. It may now be inverted without spilling much of the water, and placed on the skin where the leeches are to be applied. They will soon settle. As soon as they have taken hold, place a sponge or towel on one side of the glass to soak up the water, and remove it.

If one is required on any particular spot, a leech glass may be used, or—if you have not one at hand—a small phial may be used instead, by placing the leech in it head outwards.

The tail may be distinguished from the head by its being narrower, and by seeing in what direction the leech progresses when at liberty, as it always moves head foremost.

When leeches have taken their fill, they usually drop off; but sometimes they will stick on for a long time. In this case they should not be dragged away forcibly, as the teeth may be left in the wound; but a little salt applied to them will speedily cause them to relax their hold.

The quantity of blood obtained by one leech is estimated at less than a tea-spoonful ʒ i.., but this may be increased to a table-spoonful (ʒ iv.), by fomentation with warm water.

To stop bleeding, the pressure of the finger, or of a small pad of lint, for a few minutes (especially if the leeches are over a bony surface, as they should be in children), usually suffices; but if this fail and the bleeding persist, a little tincture of iron diluted, or a point of caustic will generally arrest it.

CUPPING.

The regular apparatus for cupping consists of cupping-glasses of two or three sizes; a scarificator, viz., a box of lancets, which are made to shoot out and return with a spring; and a spirit-torch, which is a small hollow metal globe filled with spirits of wine, and with a long tube stretching from it, containing a cotton wick, which is fed with spirit from the globe.

Add to these a basin of warm water for rinsing out the cupping-glasses; sponges, and a little strapping or sticking-plaister. Cotton wool, or tow, is also necessary, where the ward-sister does not possess a spirit-torch.

The cupping-glass to be applied should he first rinsed in warm water, rapidly dried, and then placed on the part desired with its face downwards, leaving sufficient room for the pipe of the lighted spirit-torch to enter at one side. The pipe must be held a few seconds in the glass to rarefy the air, then quickly withdrawn, and the cupping-glass as quickly brought down upon the skin, so as to apply the whole of its edge, when the skin is drawn into the glass and partly fills the vacuum created.

The glass will not fall off, the weight of the external air holding it firmly down, and it should therefore be left on in this state for two or three minutes.

To remove the glass, incline it a little on one side with one hand, whilst the thumb of the other hand presses the skin firmly near its edge, when the air rushes in, and the glass comes off.

Immediately this is done the scarificator—its lancets having been set—is to be placed with its face upon the skin which has been drawn up; and then, by touching its spring, the lancets make their cuts and return home.

The cupping-glass is now again put on, in the same way as at first and upon the same part, and very soon the blood is seen oozing up through the wounds and filling the cupping-glass more or less completely, as the vacuum is more or less perfect. If sufficient blood be not obtained at the first application of the cup or cups, they must be removed as soon as they cease to fill, the wounds wiped lightly with a sponge, and the glasses put on as before.

The wounds generally cease bleeding when the cups have been taken off, and a piece of strapping or sticking-plaister is merely put on to keep them free from dirt.

Care must be taken to hold the lighted spirit-torch in such a way that it shall not burn the skin.

Great care is necessary in the German and French methods of "cupping," as they do not use a spirit-torch, but merely throw a bit of lighted cotton-wool, or tow, into the cupping-lass to rarefy the air, before applying the glass to the skin. The tow, or cotton-wool, is immediately extinguished when turned down from want of air, but there is a slight danger of burning the skin when this method is used by an inexperienced hand.

BLISTERS.

A blister may be raised by using the ordinary blister-plaister, or by painting on a blistering fluid upon the surface.

A blister-plaister should never be applied to any part of the skin which is excoriated, or otherwise broken.

The part to be blistered should be well cleaned with a little soap and warm water, and rubbed dry with a rough towel.

A blister has commonly a margin of adhesive plaister from half-an-inch to an inch wide all round, to prevent it from slipping away from the part to which it is applied; but this is objectionable, in consequence of the dragging pain which is produced when the fluid accumulates underneath the cuticle. It is better to secure the blister in position by some cotton wadding, or a fold or two of old linen and a bandage.

A blister should not be removed until it has risen; but the time varies from six to twelve hours in different people, and in different parts of the body.

When the blister is removed before it has risen sufficiently, vesication may be completed by a hot poultice applied over the part. If a poultice is kept on over the blister plaister, the vesicle is large and less painful.

To dress a blister, first remove the plaister carefully, as the part has become very tender. The cuticle should then be snipped at the most depending part, and the serum evacuated into a small dressing-cup held to receive it. If the intention is to heal the blistered surface, it should be dressed, without removing the cuticle, with simple dressing.

If it be desirable to keep the blister "open," *i. e.*, to prevent it from healing, the cuticle should be removed by cutting it round the edge with a pair of scissors, and the resin, sabine, or mercurial ointment should then be spread upon lint and applied.

These applications must be repeated daily, after the sore has been carefully washed.

SECTION XIV.

SURGICAL, STARCHED, AND OTHER BANDAGES; SPLINT PADDING; CHAFF PILLOWS; SAND BAGS.

The best bandages for surgical purposes are made of old strong linen. They are cut by the thread the length required, and "herringboned" one end over the other, where a join is necessary.

Medical and gum bandages are usually made of unbleached calico or muslin.

For burns, flannel bandages are generally required.

The web of flannel, muslin, or calico should How made, be snipped on one selvage into the requisite breadths, and then torn across, so as to preserve the elasticity of the strips. These should be joined in the same manner as the linen bandages, until the requisite length is attained.

The selvages ought always to be stripped off, and the bandage ought, as far as possible, to be made of one continuous piece without joinings.

The common roller varies in length and width according to the part to which it is to be applied.

Arm rollers should be $2^{1}/_{8}$ inches in width, and not less than 6 yards in length.

Leg rollers should not be wider than $2\frac{1}{4}$ inches, and not less than 9 yards in length.

Rib or chest rollers should be 4½ inches wide and 12 yards long; or, 6 to 12 inches in width, and 6 to 8 yards long. They are usually made of flannel.

A number of bandages of all kinds should be kept ready for use, and arranged in a place appointed for that purpose, according to their size and quality.

It is best to use a machine for rolling bandages; for although it can be done equally well by hand, it cannot be done so quickly.

The T bandage is made by sewing two pieces of bandage of suitable length in the form of the letter T, and is used for keeping in place dressings, or other appliances, in connection with the perinæum or genital organs. The upper cross bar should be long enough to go round the waist and fasten in front, and the other to reach from the centre of the back under the perinæum and up to the waist in front. The end of the latter must be sewn to the centre of the former all across, to make it secure. The perinæal band may be left entire, or stripped into two tails which can be fastened separately over each groin.

A double-headed bandage is rolled from both ends to about the middle; or two single headed rollers may be sewn together at the free ends.

Compound bandages are formed by uniting one roller to another, or to something else, at any required angle.

Four-tailed and six-tailed bandages are made by drawing the number of threads at the required intervals, and then by carefully cutting both ends of a piece of old stout linen to within a few inches of the centre, into as many strips or tails as are desired.

Many-tailed bandages consist of a number of separate lengths of bandage linen, flannel, or calico, placed one upon the other, so that each length shall overlap the preceding one by about a third of its width. And all are then sewn to another length, placed vertically across the centre of the others.

The lengths must be cut sufficiently long to overlap each other, after encircling the part for which the bandage is intended.

A finger bandage should be about half-an-inch or an inch in width.

This bandage can be readily made by cutting an ordinary wound-up roller into two or more widths.

Ovariotomy bandages should be made of white flannel, from 30 to 40 inches in length and about one foot wide. They may have an outer covering of strong linen, to give greater support.

Two or three sets of tapes should be firmly placed at different intervals. The tapes should be at the edge of one end, and sewn 9 to 12 inches back from the edge of the other. By this means the pressure may be varied according to the size of the patient.

Triangular bandages are squares, or triangular-shaped pieces of old stout linen from 2 to 4 feet in length, measuring from corner to corner.

They are much used in Germany instead of the common roller, and certainly few of the objections made to the ordinary bandage can be applied to this.

STARCHED, AND OTHER STIFF BANDAGES.

Make a thick paste of arrowroot, or any starch other kind of starch; moisten a bandage in the paste and roll it up as an ordinary roller; then place it in the vessel of paste to get thoroughly saturated, while the limb is prepared for its application.

Dextrine, white of egg, and flour, powdered gum, and precipitated chalk may also be used for the preparation of stiff bandages.

First lay a piece of broad tape flatly along the surface on the whole length of the limb, then protect the skin completely by a narrow flannel bandage, including the heel, if the leg is the limb to be dealt with.

Apply the starched bandage in the same way as an ordinary roller, covering the surface with two layers of bandage at least, strengthening any part which may require extra support, by short strips of lint or bandage, also moistened in the paste. Some paste may now be rubbed over the bandage to ensure its having a sufficient degree of thickness.

Care must be taken that during the drying process the limb is kept in a proper position, and is not allowed to stick to the bed-clothes.

After drying, the bandage is sometimes found to be loose; it may then be slit up by means of a proper instrument (Liston's pliers), and re-applied by the addition of a common roller.

The tape first laid on the limb will be found useful in raising the bandage during the slitting-up process.

A Plaster of Paris bandage is usually made as follows:—Dust dry-powdered gypsum into the meshes of a coarse muslin bandage, and roll it up ready for use.

Envelope the limb in a flannel roller or layer of cotton-wool, soak the muslin roller, previously prepared, in water, and apply it over the flannel as an ordinary roller; then smear it over with a thick paste of gypsum and water, making the outside perfectly smooth. Keep the limb in proper position while the plaster sets, which it will in a few minutes.

Short strips of bandage are by some surgeons preferred to a roller in applying this bandage.

Flour paste or spirit varnish painted over the plaster when it has dried will prevent it chipping and keep it clean. This method is generally adopted abroad.

For gutta-percha splints cut out of a piece of long-cloth, the shape of the part to which splints, the splint is to be applied. Taking this as a pattern, cut a piece of gutta-percha of corresponding dimensions.

Have some boiling water ready in a pan, and when all is ready dip the piece of gutta-percha in the water completely for a few seconds until it has become pliable.

Take the softened gutta-percha out quickly, lay the pattern cloth upon it, to protect the skin, and apply it on the part.

It must then be rapidly moulded to it by pressure, and a roller bound over it before it hardens, that it may adapt itself closely to the surface.

Sole-leather or mill-board may be used in a similar way.

SPLINT PADDING.

Splints made of wood, tin, or japanned iron, require to be lined with some description of soft padding before application.

The sister of a ward should always keep one complete set of pads to the most commonly used splints in readiness for any emergency.

The best with which I am acquainted are those that were in use at St. Thomas's Hospital when I was in training there.

They were made of three or more thicknesses of old blankets, or woollen rugs, covered on both sides with old linen sheeting, and quilted through by running across in a large diamond pattern.

These pads will wash.

Another pad is made by teasing tow, covering it with soft muslin and quilting it in the same way as the washing pad.

The perinæal band or bandage is made of the same materials, *i.e.*, of teased tow or cotton-wool mixed, or of cotton-wool, or of tow alone.

Cut a bandage from 3 to 4 inches wide, and one and a-half yard long. The best material is old, soft, strong linen. Join it down the middle half a yard at each end, leaving the ends pointed and tapering, and padding or stuffing the centre of bandage as above.

When completed, stitch the bandage across where the padding ends, and run a thread lightly down the middle of the padding to keep it in position.

The padded part should afterwards be covered with oil-silk, gutta-percha or india-rubber cloth.

These bands may be of various sizes.

CHAFF PILLOWS.

Chaff pillows may be useful to prop a weakly patient when turned on his side, and are in frequent requisition, in surgical wards, in cases of amputation, fracture, or sprain. They should vary in size from a few inches square to that of an ordinary pillow.

Make them of long-cloth or sheeting. Cut the material of the width and double the length of the required size; fold it across and sew it up all round except a small hole, which is to be left at one corner in order to fill it.

Turn the bag inside out so as to bring the seams inside, fill it moderately full, and close the opening.

When soiled the seam can be re-opened, the chaff emptied out, and the bag washed and refilled with fresh chaff.

SAND BAGS.

Sand bags should be prepared in the same manner.

They should be made of bed-ticking, filled with clean fine sand, and covered with waterproof.

Different sizes will be necessary, varying from 1 to 4 feet in length, and from 2 to 6 inches in thickness, in proportion to their length.

SECTION XV.

PREPARATION OF BED FOR ACCIDENTS AND EMERGENCIES; AND REMOVAL OF PATIENT'S CLOTHING.

In all surgical hospitals there are certain beds reserved for Accidents. These should always be kept made up; at night the sisters should see, before leaving their wards, that the reserved beds are properly prepared for any cases that may be brought in.

Under the mattress should be placed "fracture boards," of the same length as the width of the bedstead.

These are smooth deal boards about a foot wide, placed across the bed to render it firm.

In addition to the usual bed furniture, the bed should be provided with a large sheet of waterproofing for the protection of the mattress, and a draw sheet should be placed across the middle of the bed. It may be needed there, or be used for the protection of the pillow, as the nature of the accident may require.

A change of linen for the patient should be placed on the bed.

All tight clothing about the neck should be first loosened or removed.

If the patient is unable to move any particular part of his body without pain, care should be taken to treat that part just as though the injury were known to be of a serious nature.

After placing the patient in the middle of a bed, ascertain in what part of the body he has any pain on movement; if it be about the arms or shoulders, rip up the outer seam of the coat on the injured side, as high as the shoulder, thence along the shoulder seam to the collar; if the sound arm can now be disengaged, the coat may be slipped down over the injured limb without cutting through the collar.

The waistcoat should then be cut through from the shoulder to the neck on the side of the injury, unfastened and slipped off the other side.

If the thigh or leg has sustained an injury, Thigh or the coat and waistcoat may first be removed as gently as possible, then the outer seam of the trowsers on the side of the injury should be ripped up, and the waistband cut through; so as to open them completely.

A towel or sheet should be thrown over the man to avoid exposure, and the other trowser leg drawn off by the hand passed down under the thigh from above, rather than by dragging at the ankle part; or, the patient may be carefully raised the while by an assistant.

To facilitate the removal of the shirt, the seam on the injured side may be unripped as high as may be found requisite.

In injuries of the leg and foot, the stockings or socks may be cut away; in other cases they may generally be drawn off by care without jarring the patient.

Unnecessary destruction of clothing is to be avoided on all occasions, hence the seams should be ripped in preference to cutting through the dress in any direction, and even that may only be required in exceptional cases.

The destruction of the dress must be considered, however, a matter of little importance, when compared with the chance of inflicting injury or suffering on the patient.

In all these manipulations, firmness of touch is a great advantage.

Nothing is more useless, or a cause of more suffering, than the handling of a patient in a fitful, uncertain, purposeless way. Sometimes, however, pain cannot be avoided by the most dexterous and gentle hands.

First, consider carefully what ought to be done, and then proceed to do it at once, without putting the sufferer to the torture of two or three movements where one would suffice.

SECTION XVI.

OPERATIONS.

It is usually the duty of the sister, to whose ward the patient to be operated upon belongs, to furnish the theatre with towels, sponges, hot and cold water, tins and other receptacles required. She should take care that there are plenty of towels for the surgeon's use, wash-hand basins and soap, and blankets, pillows, and a piece of waterproof sheeting for the operating table.

It is well to have a "dressing tray," *i.e.* a wooden tray with ledge round it. This sort of tray is always used in Germany, and everything required for ordinary dressings is arranged upon it, *viz.*, olive oil, ointments, lotions, and diluted carbolic acid, with saucers for them; cotton wool, tow, lint, charpie, linen compresses; linen, calico, flannel and muslin bandages of various sizes; sponges, pins; strapping and other plaister; two or more small chaff pillows; small bowls to receive discharges, and glass syringes for wounds.

The tray and contents should be covered with a cloth, or large compress.

In hospitals where Lister's method of antiseptic treatment is adopted, the requisite carbolic acid dressings, solutions, and spray apparatus are to be at hand.

To these should be added, for operations, broad and narrow tape, needles and thread, a feeder, a small bottle of sal-volatile, brandy, and drinking-water. A little ice may be required.

Some of the strapping should be cut into a fringe of long strips, varying from ½ an inch to 3 inches in width. Lint also should be cut into strips, wetted, and laid on a plate ready for use.

During the operation the sister is usually required to clean and squeeze the sponges used. They should be washed in cold water and squeezed as dry as possible, the best way being to place them in a cloth and turn the two ends rapidly in opposite ways.

The patient should be dressed as lightly as possible.

All bands about the neck and waist should invariably be loosened.

The part to be operated on should either be left uncovered, or be covered only by a loose article of dress, which can be thrown off in a moment.

The dressings should be removed, the surface of wound cleansed, and the part simply covered lightly with a piece of wet lint, or a turn or two of a roller.

If possible the patient should have a bath on the morning of the operation, or the day before, and such medical preparation as the surgeon shall direct.

If chloroform is to be used, the patient should not be permitted to take any food, except perhaps beef-tea, coffee, or other fluid, for 4 or 5 hours previous to the operation.

In all operations on or near the bladder and rectum, and in ovariotomy operations, the sister should ask for directions, as to whether an enema is to be administered the morning of the operation, and of what kind; and whether the bladder should be emptied by the catheter.

If still under the influence of chloroform after the operation, the patient should be laid on his back in a clean bed, with his head somewhat raised.

There should be no impediment to the free access of fresh air, but he should be kept warm; and, if necessary, he should have a hot-water bottle applied to his feet or body, and a stimulant should be administered if directed or permitted.

If vomiting occur he may be turned on his side, and the head held over a basin, care being taken to avoid soiling the bed; or if he cannot be turned, the head and body may generally be raised during the vomiting.

An operation case should never be left alone, until all the ligatures have come away.

He must be carefully watched, and, if any unusual depression be observed, it must be brought to the notice of the surgeon in charge at once.

After operations of all kinds the nurse must be on the alert to see if any bleeding occur, and, if the dressings become soiled by fresh blood, no time should be lost in reporting it.

Blood is most liable to escape at the lower part of a wound, therefore it is a good plan to place a clean towel in such a position that the blood, if there is any, may soak into it, so that no considerable portion can be lost without the nurse noticing it.

After most operations the patient should be prevented from frequently moving his position in bed, and in many cases all movement is absolutely forbidden. In these the nurse will have to feed the patient from a feeding-cup, and nourishment must be given in accordance with the special instructions she will receive on that point—usually small quantities at a time, and often repeated. If sickness is caused, as it often will be after chloroform, the quantities must be reduced.

Nutritive enemata are frequently ordered in lieu of nourishment by the mouth.

Sucking small pieces of ice, or taking small quantities of iced-water, or soda-water with a little brandy, or brandy alone, will often check sickness or vomiting.

The sister should ask if there be any special instructions, and also whether, in the case of retention of urine, the patient being a female, the catheter is to be used.

The nurse should be particularly observant of any change or alteration of the condition of the patient for the first few days after an operation, and lose no time in bringing it to notice.

LITHOTOMY.

Lithotomy is the operation for the removal of the stone from the urinary bladder by cutting.

A mackintosh and draw-sheet should be placed across the middle of the bed. A bolster or pillow covered with mackintosh, and a draw-sheet or large pillow-case, should be on or near the bed; and, immediately upon the arrival of patient from the theatre, should be placed under his knees in such a way as to remove all strain from the abdominal muscles.

The bed is prepared in this way also for cases of HERNIA, LITHOTRITY, OVARIOTOMY, and all abdominal operations.

The patient should be so placed in the bed that the discharges could easily be removed before they accumulate.

The nurse should carefully notice whether any fragments of stone come away, and how much urine, if any, passes through the natural opening.

Great care must be taken in the prevention of bed-sore.

The sponges applied to the wound should be constantly changed, and rinsed in cold water and carbolic acid, always being wrung out in a strong cloth as in the case of a fomentation before applying them.

LITHOTRITY.

Lithotrity is the operation of crushing a stone in the bladder.

The patient should be kept in bed, and all that the nurse would have to do in this case would be to collect and filter every drop of urine, so that any fragment of stone that may escape, can be reserved for the observation of the surgeon.

SECTION XVII.

FEVERS.

Different diseases require different modes of nursing, concerning which the medical "chef" or chief visiting physician will give directions. A good fever nurse will never experience any difficulty in carrying out his directions, for fever is a disease which runs through many and various stages, all of them depending more or less for cure upon the nursing which they receive.

The care of a fever patient upon admittance into a medical ward, does not differ in any important respect from that already recommended in the Section on "Accidents."

The bed should be provided with a mackintosh and draw-sheet, and some disinfecting fluid should be placed in saucers under it.

The patient should be carefully washed, bathed if it be permitted, provided with fresh linen, and his own linen and clothes at once sent to a place where they can be properly disinfected and cleansed.

The sister should obtain an order to have his hair cut close, if it is not to be shaved.

Where it is the sister's duty to appoint the bed for his reception, she should be careful never to place a fever patient near a patient seriously ill with any depressing disorder.

Ventilation is so important, that it is the duty of the sister of a ward personally to see that some of the windows are always open for about an inch at the top, and that the ventilators, if there are any, are used.

She should never be satisfied as to the freshness of the atmosphere, unless she can feel the air gently moving over her face, when she is still. A fire in the room acts as a ventilator.

In fever a patient lies on his back, without moving much, and although during the first week or ten days of fever he generally is not insensible, but only heavy and indifferent, yet his weakness is such that the evacuations are passed under him almost without his cognizance. Bed-sores, in this case, are very apt to arise. Directions have already been given for the prevention of bed-sore, and I will, therefore, only here add that the sister should place under him an air, water, or horse-hair circular cushion with a hole in the middle, so that the inflamed part should not be pressed upon.

Where the confinement to bed is likely to be prolonged, a water bed, if procurable, should be used.

The bed-clothes of a fever patient must be changed very frequently, and the draw-sheet as often as it is soiled.

His night-shirt should be changed daily, and oftener if required.

When frequent sponging of the body with cold or tepid water, with or without vinegar, is ordered, care should be taken that only a small portion is sponged at a time.

The sponge should be passed in only one direction, and that downwards, and care must afterwards be taken that the skin is dried, with a warm soft towel. All rubbing of the skin must be avoided. The sponging should be renewed two or three times in the day.

Where cold affusion is ordered, a patient is generally permitted to sit up. He should be stripped and a sheet thrown over him. He should then be lifted out of bed, and seated on a stool placed in a sponging bath, or empty tub.

A nurse or assistant must support him, while another nurse pours from three to five gallons of cold water, at a temperature not under 45° F., unless distinctly ordered, over the body, rapidly shampooing the body with the palm of the hand, during and after the douche.

This can be done by the assistant who supports the patient, but it is better to have a third for this purpose.

The cold water should be continued until the patient feels cold and shivering.

He should then be rapidly dried by means of a warm bath-sheet thrown over him, and by shampooing. He is to be placed in bed, and a little warm wine and water given him to aid re-action.

The cold affusion should be given at the time ordered by the physician. It is generally either at some particular stage of the fever, or in the evening.

To apply cold affusion over the head, the patient's head must be shaved, as this affusion, or douche, consists in pouring a stream of cold water from a jug or through a funnel, over the shaved head.

The patient should be raised in bed, and the head being held over an empty basin, the stream of cold water should be directed on the crown of the head, and the vessel gradually raised so as to increase the fall of the water, as much as the patient can bear.

The head should then be dried with a soft towel, but not rubbed.

When a wet compress is ordered, the moistened cloths should be thin, and gently laid over the place appointed, not pressed upon it. (For Lotions, Ice, &c., see p. 129.) The sister must see that these cloths are kept constantly moist.

To cleanse the teeth and gums, cut a small slice of lemon, and rub it gently but firmly over the teeth, tongue, and lips. Then, with a little pure cold water and a "charpie" brush, rapidly wash over the same.

A piece of wet lint or linen twisted round the tips of a pair of dressing forceps answers as well as a charpie brush, and is more readily prepared.

Where the lemon causes the lips, or gums, to bleed, the lemon may be omitted, and two washings given instead with cold water alone. The mouth may be washed with carbolic acid spray, as previously explained.

The feet and legs of the patient must be examined by the nurse's hand, from time to time, certainly not less frequently than every hour.

Where any tendency to chill is discovered, hot bottles, hot bricks, or warm flannels, with some warm drink, should be made use of until the temperature is restored.

Where a patient is too weak to brush away the flies himself, the sister should see that he is provided with a veil of gauze or muslin.

By tying strings across the bed, these veils may be supported away from the patient's face.

Nourishment and stimulant should be given at the exact time appointed by the physician: this is generally every two hours, every hour, or in bad cases every half-hour or oftener.

The sister should ask for special directions as to the time and quantity.

Stimulant is usually given in small portions at a time, mixed with barley water, or some farinaceous substance.

Even if a patient is asleep who has been without sleep for days, the nourishment or stimulant must be given at each appointed hour, or he is not unlikely to awake and pass into a state of fatal collapse.

Where opium is ordered to be administered, in cases of general irritability and sleeplessness, it is usually left to the sister to administer it at certain prescribed intervals until the patient is calmed.

In remittent fever it must be remembered that quinine is given in smaller doses when the fever is high, than during the remission.

When delirium sets in, the nurse must increase her watchfulness, for, it has been truly said, the patient depends for very life itself upon her conscientious care.

Never contradict delirious patients, nor attempt to argue with them.

A nurse should avoid all roughness in dealing with them. She should be firm in dealing with them, and, although she should endeavour to appear interested in their conversation, should never allow herself to tell an untruth. A patient must never see that a nurse is afraid of him, or inclined to let him have his own way.

A nurse should never be left alone with a patient in delirium, unless immediate assistance is available at a moment's notice.

Every contrivance must be employed to save the patient's strength during the first stage of convalescence.

Pillows of different forms and sizes should be so placed as to prop the body into the most comfortable positions for the time.

The patient should not be allowed to feed himself, and where solid food is allowed, it should be minced and given him in a spoon.

The Sœurs de Charité in the Military Hospital of the Val-de-Grâce always pinned a clean towel round the neck of the patient they were feeding. This kept the patient's linen clean, and prevented the bedclothes being soiled in any way. They also always gave fresh water and the patient's hand-towel after each meal, to patients who were unable to rise and wash in the lavatory.

They exercised the utmost ingenuity to amuse and interest patients at this stage, bringing them fresh flowers, pictures, and the like.

It is at this period that the skill of the sister must be exercised in varying the prescribed hospital diet, as much as possible.

A physician will sometimes more readily give an order for extras, such as milk and eggs, if there is any place for cooking them attached to the ward.

SECTION XVIII.

ERUPTIVE FEVERS.

The most common and the most to be dreaded of all fevers attended with eruption, is small-pox.

Small-pox is rarely admitted into our general hospitals, but it is common in our workhouse infirmaries, and a sister or superintendent of such an infirmary may have to instruct her nurses and probationers how to nurse such cases.

It is well to bear in mind that there is no antidote or medicine to cut short the disease; all that can be done is to guide the patient safely through it. A full supply of fresh air is most essential. In many instances, temporary huts and tents have therefore proved to be excellent hospitals.

The rules given in the section on fevers with regard to the admittance of patients, ventilation, protection from flies, and keeping the extremities warm, and delirium, should also be followed in eruptive fevers.

For the early stages when the skin is very hot, tepid sponging will prove refreshing, especially if its use be followed by a change of linen. It was not permitted, however, by any medical man under whom I worked in France; but the eyes and nostrils were cleansed with water and a little charpie brush or morsel of lint as often as required. When the pustules have burst, this is all that is practicable.

In confluent cases, the head should be shaved early, or the hair cut very closely, otherwise matting of the hair will take place.

Early application of light poultices to the face have been found a great comfort, and an almost certain protective against "pitting."

The bed should be arranged with mackintosh, and draw-sheet, as for fever; but the coverings should be light woollen blankets, and no counterpane of cotton permitted.

Where there is the least fear of the occurrence of ulceration on the back or nates, the patient should be placed on a water-bed, or on one of Hooper's large water-pillows.

The usual remedies against bed-sore cannot be used.

The sheets and night-shirt of the patient Linen, should be changed daily; the draw-sheet as often as required.

All linen must be warmed, as well as aired.

Cooling drinks, such as imperial ice-water, barley-water, raspberry vinegar and water, lemonade, and soda-water, are grateful to the patient, and should be given him every half-hour or oftener.

In raising a patient to drink, the left hand should be placed under the pillow of the patient, and the head and the pillow lifted together, taking care that the head is straight, that the drink may not run from the corners of the lips.

In *primary fever*, the diet usually consists of arrowroot, gruel, weak beef-tea, tea with milk, and ripe fruits.

In *secondary fever*, strong beef-tea, good soup, milk or cream, the yolk of one or two eggs daily, are probably ordered.

Where stimulants are ordered, the directions given under "Fevers" should be followed.

A sister or nurse in an English hospital has nothing to do with prescribing medicines, or ordering stimulants, but in many of our large workhouse infirmaries more is left to the discretion and knowledge of the superintendent, sisters, and nurses, than is usual in general hospitals, to which there is generally attached a large staff of medical men.

To allay the itching, oil the pustules on the face, neck, and hands with olive oil, glycerine, cold cream, or officinal lime liniment, according to the order given. A large camel-hair paint-brush should be used, or a brush made of charpie. In the French hospitals we always used olive oil.

Care must be taken that all folds of the skin are well oiled; such as, for instance, those between the face and neck, and behind the ears.

If the eruption seems unable to appear on hard surfaces, such as soles of feet, knees, or palms of hands, apply linseed poultices until the skin is sufficiently softened for them to rise well.

In *secondary fever*, or when the pustules disappear, watch carefully whether there is any increase of fever, rapid pulse, &c., as this time complications are apt to arise, and should be promptly treated.

The sister, or nurse, must examine the body carefully, and, if she finds any signs of abscess forming, or already formed, should apply linseed poultices to them, and mention it to the physician or surgeon at his next visit.

When the pustules have burst, some dry powder—as the oxide of zinc or powdered starch, is often freely applied to absorb the matter.

The eruption of pimples or papulæ always begins to show itself on the third day of the fever.

The papulæ gradually ripen into pustules, the suppuration being complete by the ninth day, when the pustules break, and crusts or scabs are formed.

In four or five days more these scabs begin to fall off.

About this time a patient is generally so far convalescent that a bath is frequently ordered.

Great care must be taken that he be not chilled.

It is almost needless to add that the exposure of a small-pox patient to the company of persons not infected is both immoral and illegal.

Small-pox is communicable by contact with the affected, through the air, or by fomites—by which is meant any material to which the poison can adhere, such as clothes, bedding, furniture, bales of cotton, or ships. As a rule, one attack of small-pox will render a person insusceptible to a second attack. I may add, that I never saw one death from this disease where several vaccination scars were well marked.

SECTION XIX.

ANTISEPTICS AND DISINFECTANTS.

There is still considerable doubt as to the mode of action, and therefore as to the relative value of some of these substances. For practical purposes the chief of them may be classed under two heads:

First, those employed in occupied wards; and *second*, those used for disinfection of empty contagious wards.

Under the first head are included Condy's fluid, Carbolic acid, Chloralum.

(*a*) CONDY'S FLUID is a strong solution of the permanganate of potash, which, more or less diluted, is exposed in vessels scattered through a ward.

(*b*) CARBOLIC ACID in solution, or in the form of McDougall's disinfecting powder, may be sprinkled over a ward, or the former may be placed in exposed vessels, like Condy's fluid.

(c) CHLORALUM may be similarly used.

Under the second head are included Chlorine gas and Sulphurous acid gas.

(*d*) CHLORINE GAS. As a fumigating antiseptic and disinfectant, chlorine gas is said to stand unrivalled. The ingredients for producing it should be contained in saucers placed in the higher parts of the ward. It may be produced thus:—One part of common salt intimately mixed with one part of the black, or binoxide of, manganese, placed in a shallow earthen pan; two parts of oil of vitriol, previously diluted with two parts by measure of water, should then be poured over it, and the whole stirred with a stick. Chlorine will continue to be liberated from this mixture for four days. It is necessary while employing it that the doors, windows, and chimney of the room be kept carefully closed for some hours.

(b) SULPHUROUS ACID GAS. The most convenient and cheapest means of disinfecting a ward, with its contents in the way of furniture, is to expose it to the action of this gas.

All windows and doors of the ward should be closed while a stick of brimstone is burnt within, so as to fill the chamber with the fumes. This done, the doors and windows are opened, and McDougall's powder sprinkled on the floor, while the cots and furniture should be washed with a solution of carbolic acid, one part of the crystals in twenty parts of water.

THE END.

www.ingramcontent.com/pod-product-compliance
Lightning Source LLC
Chambersburg PA
CBHW070252190526
45169CB00001B/376